S0-BUF-954

HELPING CHRONICALLY ILL CHILDREN IN SCHOOL

A Practical Guide for Teachers, Counselors, and Administrators

Gertrude Morrow
Certified School Psychologist

ASU WEST LIBRARY

LC
4545
.m66
1985
WEST

A15021 966309

Parker Publishing Company, Inc.   **West Nyack, New York**

© 1985 *by*

PARKER PUBLISHING COMPANY, INC.

West Nyack, N.Y.

All rights reserved. No part of this
book may be reproduced in any form or
by any means, without permission in
writing from the publisher.

Library of Congress Cataloging in Publication Data

Morrow, Gertrude.
  Helping chronically ill children in school.

  Bibliography: p.
  Includes index.
  1. Chronically ill children—Education.   2. Hospital
schools.   3. Chronically ill children—Family
relationships.   4. Home and school.   I. Title.
LC4545.M66   1985   371.9   85-19245

ISBN 0-13-386053-1

Printed in the United States of America

For my children,
Suzan, Jeffry, Rebecca, Gregory, Harry, and Trudy

ACKNOWLEDGMENTS

I would like to thank the people who have given me support and encouragement, as well as helpful suggestions during the writing of this book. My pediatrician husband William was always available as a medical consultant and also shared with me his dilemmas over chronically ill patients and their families. Fellow staff members of school district #28, Northbrook, Illinois, were able to point me in new directions when I felt stuck. Among those who were especially interested are Superintendent Homer Harvey, Dr. James Kucienski, Joellen Mack, Lynn Moore, Elizabeth Tremulis, Helen McPherson, Joan Grauer, Jean Merzon, Irene Lane, and Mabel Janke. My former colleagues at Evanston Hospital were most reinforcing of my efforts, and their encouragement was heartwarming. Dr. Carol Ceithaml, Dr. Gloria Berkwits, Roger Silverstein, Nora Mañago, and Dr. Lee Karon deserve particular mention. My good friend Dr. Christine San José was both educational consultant and literary critic. She read the manuscript in its early draft, and her critique was most valuable. Another friend, Dr. Joann Bentley Hoeppner, who is a neuropsychologist, read and gave a critique of Chapter 5, checking for accuracy. She also wrote the explanation of seizures contained in that chapter. My heartfelt thanks to everyone.

ABOUT THIS BOOK

Helping Chronically Ill Children in School was written to assist the teacher, counselor, and school administrator in handling the special problems of the chronically ill student.

Advances in medicine and medical research have enabled more chronically ill children to attend school. Therefore, although their overall number is small (10 to 15 percent of the school population), more and more teachers are encountering these children and attempting to meet their special needs.

Having been a chronically ill child myself, I have a special empathy for these children and am sensitive to their needs in a school setting. My personal experiences are described in Chapter 1.

If chronic illness has been diagnosed before children enter kindergarten, starting school will be more stressful for them than for the usual child. Chapter 2 discusses the importance of planning and being prepared to meet a wide range of exigencies that may present themselves. The teacher will learn how to deal with common separation problems and what to do when an ill child suddenly becomes upset in school.

Chronically ill children feel that they are different from others, even when there is no external evidence of their difference. Teachers play a significant role in helping such children recognize that, in most ways, they are the same as other children. Teachers can also help chronically ill children to cope, to feel okay about themselves, and to believe in their worth as human beings. Teachers can create an atmosphere in the classroom that fosters the ill child's acceptance by other children. Chapters 3, 4, and 5 discuss these issues.

When a chronically ill child is having trouble learning, analyzing the basis of the problem is the first step toward finding a solution. In Chapter 6, the teacher will be shown how to analyze a learning problem and what to do about it.

Teachers have a role to play in helping a child prepare for hospitalization and in making the transition back to school as smooth and pleasant as possible. They can guide parents in how to give support to the child, can maintain contact with the child in the hospital, and can communicate the child's needs to the home/hospital teacher. These topics are discussed in Chapter 7.

Many important ways teachers can indirectly help ill children involve relationships. Siblings are deeply affected by having a brother or sister who is chronically ill, and how teachers can help is discussed in Chapter 8.

The teacher is also in a position to give guidance to parents. By understanding the impact of a child's illness on the family and how the family can successfully cope, the teacher can give appropriate guidance. Chapter 9 points the way toward helping these families deal with their situation.

Teachers need to find ways to reestablish and maintain rapport with parents if barriers develop between the home and the school. When they have a good relationship with the ill child's doctor, they may find the doctor can help in resolving conflicts between them and the parent. Chapter 10 deals with barrier removal and how to develop a relationship with a child's doctor.

Teachers are responsible for guiding parents toward using whichever special services the school has to offer. Chapters 11 and 12 provide the teacher with information about the roles of special staff members, the components of a Child Study Evaluation, and the rights of parents. Parental fears and worries over psychological evaluation, counseling, and special classes are discussed so that the teacher will know how to gain parental acceptance and to get permission to actively lend a hand.

What the future holds for chronically ill children will be determined by how well teachers learn to work with parents and other professionals. As allies, these significant adults have the power to enrich the life of chronically ill children and to help them achieve optimal development. The challenge of becoming partners with parents and other professionals will best be met if teachers understand the others' roles, responsibilities, and realities, and work with them from a position of equality. Chapter 13 provides techniques for attaining ideal relationships between parents, teachers, and doctors.

Throughout this book, you will meet many real children (although their names have been changed) in brief vignettes portraying particular problems they have had to face. As you meet them, you will learn how to give your chronically ill students the kind of help they need to ease their adjustment at school and at home, and to promote their psychological and intellectual growth.

Gertrude Morrow

CONTENTS

WHAT IT MEANS TO BE CHRONICALLY ILL: MY OWN EXPERIENCE AS A CHILD

I believe that a teacher should start by trying to enter the inner world of a chronically ill child. By presenting a personal account of my own struggles as a child who was chronically ill, I hope that teachers will get an understanding for what a child experiences, for the problems and dilemmas that must be faced by the child and the family, and for the importance of a compassionate and caring teacher.

PAINFUL BEGINNINGS

My illness started on the first day of school in the fall of 1928. People were not psychologically sophisticated in those days, but intuitively they assumed that the severe pain that I complained of in my leg was only in my imagination—a result of being afraid of school.

The illness I had, osteomyelitis, was a chronic recurring infection of the bone. The danger of fatal blood poisoning was great. This illness can now be treated with antibiotics, but fifty years ago the treatment was surgical. I was a child who went from school to hospital and back again before the era of hospital playrooms and child-life specialists, of school psychological services and special education programs.

Medically, I experienced major operations that left mutilating scars, recurrence of the illness without warning, and episodes of being on the brink of death. Psychologically, I felt fear of the next hospitalization, mounting anxiety as the surgeries became more radical, and humiliation when bodily functions and emotions were not controlled.

I had to go to school on crutches, wearing a cast with an offensive odor from the draining infection it enclosed, shunned by children, and feeling dependent on an older sister, who was not always readily available.

HOSPITAL LIFE

I have only a few memories of my several hospitalizations. The loneliness was great. Day after day, from my window, I would watch children playing on the hospital lawn and yearn to be with them. The hospital had a children's ward, but most of the time I was in a private room and had no contact with children for months at a time. Parental visiting in the children's ward was limited to once a week, a common practice in hospitals until the 1960s. Toward the end of my last hospitalization, I was moved to the children's ward. The doctors had convinced my parents that I needed children more than I needed parents at that time, and I am sure they were right.

I recall two toys that must have had some therapeutic value in my psychological coping. One toy was a huge clown balloon with cardboard feet. When it was thrown into the air, it always landed on its feet. I identified with this toy, gaining some sense of mastery and joy from it. I knew I must keep smiling (as the clown did) despite everything, and I hoped *I* would end up on *my* feet. The other toy was a mechanical one. Circus acrobats swung, twirled, or went over the top on their trapezes when the toy was wound up, only gradually coming to a stop as the mechanical part ran down. Wasn't my illness like their actions: swinging back and forth between sickness and health? There was a vicarious thrill in watching glorious movements I could not engage in. The fact that I could control the actions of the acrobats (by winding, or refusing to wind) was perhaps a symbolic replacement of the control I no longer had in regard to my own body and actions.

BACK TO SCHOOL

After surgeries, hospitalization, and home recuperation, my return to school was planned. The educational dilemma centered on where I should be placed in school. I had missed the second semester of first grade (I had started at midyear) and was not ready for second grade. By coincidence, the school had decided to open a special class for children who had failed to learn to read. I was placed in this class.

Everyone knew that the kids in the special room were not bright, and I felt the stigma of being thought of as a dummy. However, despite the fact that I felt humiliation and shame at the time, and have perhaps overcompensated in regard to intellectual pursuits all my life, there were positive aspects to the experience for me. I felt challenged to get out of that class and worked hard at learning to read. As there were only seven children in the class, I had lots of loving care and attention from my teacher. Who knows whether I would have been motivated without this?

I was never again in a special class. Later, after a critical bout of my illness, when I was on crutches for a long time, consideration was given to whether I should be moved to the local school for crippled children. This was vetoed, and, being a child, I was not privy to the reasons why. I remember that I wanted to go to the special school. The physical struggles of moving from class to class in a three-story building while on crutches—and the anguish of feeling shunned and rejected—were so great that I knew I would have been more comfortable in a building designed for the physically handicapped and used by other children on crutches or in wheelchairs.

GROWING UP

During periods when I was well, my behavior was bad. I did not know how to get along with children because I had had little chance to learn. I had become ill at six and a half, the age when children begin to learn to play in groups, and according to rules. During this crucial stage in school-age social development, I was periodically isolated in the hospital. I wanted to be a boy. Boys could wear pants, which would cover my scarred leg, and boys could be tough, which I felt I had to be. I got into fights or joined others in acts of scapegoating. I had emotional explosions followed by crying from the shame of having lost control.

At about age ten, my doctor predicted that I would have no further bouts of the illness because of the success of the latest radical surgery. At this time, my physical and social rehabilitation was begun. Because my lack of physical skills was a source of embarrassment to me, gym class was the most dreaded part of the day. I could neither jump rope nor ride a bike, and I was very awkward in using playground equipment.

My family responded to my plight. My father built me a playground-size swing set, and my brother taught me to ride a bike. Then it was up to me. With persistent practice, I began to acquire skills that my peers had attained several years earlier. I was also launched into a program of structured social and recreational activities that, within a few years, helped me to emerge from being socially maladjusted.

Although I was the usual skinny, gawky pre-teenager and not a thing of beauty, I had the potential to become a reasonably attractive female except for my "bad leg." As the leg was both bowed and se-verely scarred, my mother found ways, within the accepted style of the day, to hide the scar. This was done to protect me from the stares of others, but I understood that others should not be offended by the sight of it.

My mother wanted me to enjoy the pleasure of swimming, and this meant that I had to cope with exposing the scar. I learned that, although one kind of exposure was acceptable, another was not. I could swim and play sports, but I couldn't take tap dancing as my sister did. The scarred leg would spoil the beauty of a chorus line of ten-year-olds, but wouldn't bother anyone in the swimming pool.

The scarred leg interfered with my accepting myself as a feminine person. I persisted in denying my interest in boys until after a plastic surgery operation at age eighteen transformed the very ugly scar into a quite acceptable one. Throughout this period, I dared, in my private world, to imagine myself when grown as a glamorous nightclub singer, sought after by men. My beautiful evening gowns would conceal the ugly scar. This fantasy was most useful to me because it helped me maintain hope in becoming a normal female.

FAMILY SUPPORT

My siblings played an important part in my growing up success-fully. A younger brother was a pal to me during my tomboy years. An older brother let me try out feminine silliness on him. My relationship with my sister, just a year older than I, was more difficult for me. We were often perceived as twins, and I was expected to do things at the same time that she was ready. However, my sister was also assigned to be my mother-protector. This was a mixed blessing. Having her in this role gave me the needed security to venture into many experiences I might otherwise have avoided, but it also reinforced a sense of depen-dency. It was somewhat of a strain, and also confusing, that at one moment I was expected to perform on a par with Marjorie and simul-taneously experience what she was ready for, and then, at the next moment I was considered helpless, dependent, and in need of her protection.

My parents intuitively did the right things most of the time. The only thing they did not realize was that I was not always emotionally ready for some experiences, and their timing was sometimes a bit off. I would have felt less pressured if I had not been expected to catch up to my peers in *everything* so fast.

Although my family assumed most of the responsibility for my rehabilitation, they did so by working cooperatively with the school. In today's world, many families are not able to provide the kind of rehabilitation needed, and teachers are more important than ever to special children.

In the chapters that follow, the role of the teacher in handling specific situations and problems of the chronically ill child are discussed.

2

STARTING SCHOOL: PLANNING AND PREPARING TO MEET SPECIAL NEEDS

> It is mid-August and Mrs. Barber is feeling anxious and upset. Her daughter, Karen, is supposed to start school soon, and she can't force herself to think about it. How can she send her sick little girl to school when she has so much pain every day and needs a lot of comforting and reassurance?

When chronic illness has been diagnosed in infancy or during the preschool years, starting school will be a major trauma. Many mothers will feel as torn and ambivalent as Mrs. Barber. Wise mothers will become acquainted with the school staff long before the opening day of kindergarten. They will schedule conferences with the school nurse and principal the spring before, and they will ask permission to visit the kindergarten classes. The more that the school staff knows about the child's medical experience and about the child's reactions to her illness, the better prepared they will be to meet her needs and deal with problems that arise. This chapter discusses the common problems a teacher may encounter with a chronically ill pupil. Ways to deal with exigencies that arise will be considered here.

APPROPRIATE TIME TO START SCHOOL

A great many children are not ready to start school at the time that state law says they may enter. Research indicates that children will have a much greater chance of being successful in school if they are five years old or older before starting kindergarten. When a child has encountered serious medical problems during his early years, it is even more crucial that he should not begin school before he has had his fifth birthday. It is possible that many younger children can make an adequate adjustment to kindergarten, particularly if they have attended a preschool program. However, the younger children may not be emotionally ready the following year to respond to the demands of first grade, or they may not be mature enough to meet the behavioral standards of first grade. The curriculum in many schools has been drastically accelerated. Children are introduced to reading readiness in kindergarten. In first grade, they are expected to cover what was, a generation ago, a second grade curriculum. The accelerated pressure continues throughout the school years. Teachers and administrators know this, but parents usually do not. This is the reason a principal or other school person who is consulted should advise them to wait, when parents ask if they should start their not-yet-five-year-old child in school.

SEPARATION DIFFICULTY WHEN STARTING SCHOOL

There is a strong tendency for mother and child to become intensely bound to each other when the child has a serious illness. When it comes time to start school, a mother may have trouble letting go. Giving her child over to the authority and influence of the teacher will be hard. The child will sense this pull from the mother and try to stay close to her.

Almost all children have some degree of separation anxiety upon starting kindergarten, even if they don't show it.[1] The heavy doors are hard to open; there are swarms of big, noisy, aggressive kids; and the numerous rules and expectations are new, different from anything they have experienced before. Who will protect them? Who will understand that they can't do everything right all at once?

Separation difficulty is a two-sided problem. Mother is not sure her child can get along without her, and she is not sure she can get along without the child. This uncertainty combined with anxiety about whether she has been a good mother and ambivalence about whether the child is ready, or psychologically self-sufficient to get along without her are dynamics of separation difficulty. The child reacts to the mother's ambivalence and uncertainty, often without realizing it, by behaviors that communicate that he indeed wishes and needs to be at home with his mother. If the mother does not have confidence in the child's ability to stand on his own two feet, how can he? If the mother thinks the child will not be safe at school, away from her attentive care, how can he feel safe?

Separation anxiety in a chronically ill child is likely to be very emotionally charged because the illness has made the child feel overly dependent and in need of protection, and has intensified the mother's protective impulses. If the child has been hospitalized during the preschool years without having a parent always available, his fear of abandonment will be more intense.

Allowing the Mother to Become a Room Helper

It is most advisable to allow the mother to stay in the kindergarten room with her fearful chronically ill child until he becomes familiar with the teacher, children, and routines. The mother's stay can gradually decrease in length until she no longer needs to stay. This may take only a few days, but it could take several weeks. The effect on other children is usually quieting. They all *wish* to have their mothers there, and somehow when one child's mother is present, all the children feel more secure. There is little danger that they will all want the same privilege. The teacher does not need to offer the class an explanation unless the children raise questions. At this age, children are convinced that all illnesses can be caught,[2] so it is best not to focus on the fact that a child is sick. The teacher can mention that this child needs his mother there, and that she can help the teacher and the children.

The mother must not be made to feel embarrassed or ashamed about being a regular visitor in the classroom. When the sick child sees the teacher and mother as allies, he will be more quickly reassured that the teacher will help and protect him in his mother's absence. After the mother has worked along with the teacher, she also should come to feel that her child is in good hands although away from her.

Reading Stories

Another way to help a child is to have the mother read stories that deal with the issue of separation. The teacher may also want to read such stories to the class. Two that are appropriate for young children are Charlotte Steiner's *I'd Rather Stay with You* (Seabury Press, NY, 1963) and Jane Thayer's *A Drink for Little Red Diker* (William Morrow, NY, 1963).[3]

SCHOOL AVOIDANCE IN OLDER CHILDREN

When a child who has been attending school for a few years develops a resistance to going, the separation anxiety is sometimes called *school phobia* or *school avoidance*. These terms mean the same thing: worry, anxiety, or fear about being in school and separated from the mother. A chronically ill child's school phobia may be caused by a feared or perceived worsening of her condition. She may be worrying about imminent medical procedures or expected surgery. (When a child has a life-threatening illness, normal separation anxiety is exacerbated by fear of the ultimate separation—death.) Once the results of tests, procedures, or surgery assure her that she's all right, the child's anxiety will usually diminish sufficiently so she no longer fears being in school.[4]

When it has been ascertained that the ill child's school avoidance is related to what's going on with her illness, she should not be forced to go to school (as is the normal procedure with well children who want to avoid school). If she cannot be gotten there with encouragement, the teacher should allow her schoolbooks to be taken home, should list her assignments, and should let the child work at home during this temporary period of anxiety. Ideally, the child should have homebound tutoring during this period; that is, the school absence should be viewed as an episode of illness. However, unless schools have a liberal policy governing homebound help, school-funded tutoring may not be granted. Regardless of what he understands to be the policy, the teacher should advise the parent to request homebound tutoring from the administration. Some states (Illinois is a case in point) have liberalized policies of paying for tutoring for chronically ill children who are frequently absent. In such a state, a child who has a documented chronic illness does not have to be absent two weeks before receiving homebound instruction at the school's expense.

PLANNING FOR SPECIAL NEEDS

A preentrance conference between the parents and the school principal is most important if a child has special needs that must be given special consideration. If the parents don't realize they should do this, perhaps a teacher, physician, or friends will have advised them to do so.

It is the principal's job to make sure that children are safe while they are in school. Information about the illness and preparation for emergencies are essential if the principal is to carry out this mandate. The principal needs to know what physical restrictions have been placed on the child and whether there are any specific dietary or medication requirements during school hours. Agreement will have to be reached about where the medicine will be kept and who will supervise the child in taking it. In this instance, the principal's authority must be respected. The principal must implement school policy and enforce rules established by the board of education and superintendent. School systems vary in their rules about taking medication in school. The principal will let the parents know what their school system's rules are.

Any special toileting needs must be discussed. If there are things a child cannot do without help, these will need to be clearly spelled out. The principal may feel it is important to talk directly with the child's doctor. In this case, the parents will be asked to grant written permission for such communication. It will help the principal to know when the doctor is usually available for phone calls. Special circumstances, such as fire drills, must be discussed if the child has serious physical restrictions or shouldn't be kept in a cramped-up position (as in a disaster drill). If the child is expected to be excused from school for visits to the doctor, physical therapy, or other treatments, the school rules about leaving school or coming late must be explained.

DECISIONS ABOUT CLASS PLACEMENT

The principal decides in whose class a child will be placed. If there are two or more classes at each grade level, the principal has a choice about where to place a chronically ill child, and the decision about class placement should be based on the qualities of the teachers. An ill or handicapped child should be placed with the teacher who is most likely to be accepting, kindly, and objective about his special needs. The teacher should be a firm but flexible person who is mature and experienced in dealing with parents. Parents of chronically ill children are often overprotective; they may infantilize their child or be overly restrictive. They may be angry, with a potential to project their anger onto the teacher. The teacher very often will have to deal with emotionality, which can be irrational in child, or parent, or both.

When the principal knows something of a teacher's personal situation, this can be helpful. Has she had a chronically ill spouse, parent, or sibling? Has she had a seriously ill child of her own? Experience with illness can produce empathy and compassion or aloofness and negativism. What has this teacher's experience done to her? Some teachers can handle the limitations of a child with cerebral palsy or the implications of a child with epilepsy, but will feel distress if a student has a life-threatening illness such as cancer. Some teachers are not bothered by physical disfigurement while others are. One teacher might deal with medical emergencies calmly while another would panic. Teachers, like all humans, have their vulnerabilities and levels of tolerance. Chronically ill children can try a teacher's patience with their fears, demands, or unpredictable emotional eruptions.

Placing a child with an accepting teacher is important for several reasons. A teacher who displays kindness and empathy and has a helping and accepting attitude will generate similar behaviors and attitudes from the other students. Children learn to be caring, altruistic, and helpful by imitating the responses of significant adults.[5] The psychological distress of the chronically ill child who is feeling different, or not so attractive, will be somewhat alleviated when he experiences acceptance.

Parents are most likely to be open with and to feel positive toward a teacher whom they perceive as accepting of their child. Parents can retreat from their tendencies to be overprotective when they know the teacher will not be rejecting, oversolicitous, too tough, or too easy on their child. Parents are grateful when they see that the teacher is getting the class to understand and accept their child. They can be at ease in working with the teacher because they do not fear that the teacher will judge or criticize their parenting.

The beginning of rapport between parents and school can take place when the principal has made the wisest decision possible in selecting a teacher who will work well with both the child and the parent.

PARENTS' CONCEALMENT OF CHILDREN'S ILLNESS

Occasionally parents will conceal their child's illness. They may have been advised to do so by their physician. Bad experiences with negative or rejecting teachers can cause a doctor to give such advice to parents. Epilepsy is a condition that is frequently concealed, by failing to report that it exists. In other instances, the facts may be distorted. For example, a child with leukemia that is in remission may be listed on the health form as having anemia, or a child with mild cerebral palsy may be reported to be a clumsy child.[6] In most cases, it is a fear of how their child will be treated that prompts parents to conceal facts. Parents are less likely to do this when there is a high degree of trust and confidence between themselves and the school staff.

It is not in the child's best interest to conceal his condition. Concealment signals to the child that his condition is something to be feared or ashamed of. Principals and teachers will certainly be offended when they learn the truth, and this will undercut the level of mutual trust that is important to maintain. The parents' anxiety may be temporarily eased by not telling the school staff about their child's disorder, but both parent and child will benefit most, in the long run, from openness and honesty.

TEACHER'S NEED FOR SUPPORT

The principal, nurse, and counselor are persons who can listen to the teacher's concerns and give reassurance as it is needed. They can also offer guidance, be used as resources, or help solve specific problems.

From the Principal

A principal's job is to give support, guidance, and supervision to teachers and other staff. No matter how carefully he considers and then selects the teacher most suited for the ill or handicapped child, he will need to offer a great deal of support to her throughout the year. The principal will need to be sure that the teacher is properly informed about the medical condition.

From the Nurse

The nurse can provide the teacher with facts about the illness to increase the teacher's understanding of the child. Knowing there is a nurse available to deal with any emergency that might arise is very reassuring to a teacher. If the school does not have a nurse on the staff, the principal will need to gain access to medical information and nursing services (perhaps through a public health department) for the teacher. Teachers should expect these things of their principal and must request them if they are not offered spontaneously.

From the Counselor

Depending on the type of illness or disability and the degree of adjustment difficulties, a teacher's frustrations, worries, and dilemmas can become severe. The counselor is someone to share her feelings with.

TEACHER'S RELATIONSHIP WITH PARENTS

Parents are often confused and contradictory in their expectations of the teacher. They may want their child treated the same as other children and, at the same time, they may expect the teacher to give the child special treatment. Parents are usually oblivious to the contradiction. They may become angry at the teacher when only one part of the expectation is met. When a parent becomes angry at the teacher, the teacher must have a buffer. The principal is the one expected to serve this role. Perhaps the principal can involve the school counselor and establish ongoing counseling for the parents. Parents are usually ashamed of having made an angry attack on the teacher, and will need to restore self-esteem. The teacher is usually shaken by the experience and needs reassurance. When anger is quickly resolved, barriers do not develop. The experience of working out misunderstandings can provide a basis for solving future differences with less tension. (See Chapter 10.)

SPECIAL NEEDS IN THE CLASSROOM

Medical Emergencies

The teacher must know what to do if a chronically ill child becomes acutely ill. Both the parents and the principal, along with the school nurse and the child's doctor, must assume some responsibility for instructing a teacher about this. Ready availability of emergency phone numbers (doctor, parent, medical rescue unit) is a must. Any emergency provisions, such as Life Savers for the diabetic or an Epi Pen Auto-Injector kit for the child who is allergic to bee stings, must be at hand. The teacher must be ready to reassure the rest of the class if an emergency arises.

It is beyond the scope of this book to explain how to deal with all the common medical emergencies that may arise. The teacher should know what to do for the specific illness a particular child has. Her main duty is to get the child help, explain to the class what happened, and reassure them. After the ill child has been taken care of, the teacher should let the children ask questions. She should also let them express what they felt, and talk about the thoughts that went through their minds. In this way, anxieties will be dealt with immediately, and any misconceptions in a child's mind about what happened can be corrected.

Teachers must remain calm in an emergency situation. This is easier said than done. To be prepared to handle a medical emergency, it is wise to have imagined ahead of time what could happen for the particular ill child in this class, and the words and actions that would be necessary. Once an appropriate scenario has been imagined, the teacher should privately rehearse the dialogue and sequence of actions, and perhaps even write them down. Once a pattern for handling the emergency has been formulated and rehearsed, it will be stored in memory in case of need.

Planning for Fire Drills

The teacher must know what special requirements are to be adhered to if there is a fire drill. If Mary is wheelchair bound, who is to push her, and should she be pushed out first or last? Can Johnny, who walks very slowly with braces, be lifted out of a window so he has more time to proceed to a safe place? What about a disaster drill? Can the child with juvenile rheumatoid arthritis remain in a doubled-up position, or is she to be allowed to stand? If it is a multilevel building and children are expected to evacuate to the basement, what is the arrangement for the wheelchair child? These things must be thought through in advance by the administration, and the teacher must be duly instructed.

Special Toileting Needs

Some children may have unusual bathroom needs. Children who have a medical problem that renders them incontinent require special consideration. In one school, a plan for such a child was worked out by the teacher and mother in a way that respected the child's wishes and supported his need to feel as grown up as possible.

Here is how Glenn's problem was handled.

> Seven-year-old Glenn had no voluntary control of bladder function, but he objected to wearing a padded diaper panty. It was decided that he would wear navy blue polyester trousers so that if he wet, it would not show and would dry quickly. The teacher, Glenn, and his mother also agreed that the teacher should send him to the bathroom every two hours to empty his bladder. With this plan, Glenn seldom wet his pants.

Some comparable plan may need to be made for a child who ambulates slowly and with difficulty. Such a child could probably not get to the bathroom fast enough if he waited until he needed to go. Teachers and mothers should come up with a favorable plan for a child. The child himself should also be asked to suggest ideas.

Children with sickle cell disease are expected to drink large amounts of water and will need to use the bathroom frequently. The diabetic child may also have urgent bathroom needs. The child with cystic fibrosis has frequent and unpleasant-smelling stools. It can save him embarrassment if he is allowed to use a bathroom in the nurse's office. Whatever the special problem, any unusual bathroom needs must be considered and planned for.

Knowing When to Show Concern

Teachers should have sufficient knowledge about a particular child's illness so they can recognize symptoms when they develop. The diabetic child who starts to have an insulin reaction must receive glucose, in some form, immediately. The teacher should have Life Savers, Coke syrup, or the like at her fingertips. The child with oligoarticular-type juvenile rheumatoid arthritis (JRA) must receive prompt attention if he begins to have visual difficulty. Iridocyclitis, an inflammation of the iris and of the muscle that controls the lens of the eye, can lead to blindness if it is not treated early. If a child with JRA complains that light hurts his eyes—or if he has red eyes or rubs his eyes a lot—he should have an eye examination without delay.[7] Parents should know this, but they will expect the teacher to report symptoms. If a teacher is uncertain about whether or not symptoms are serious, she should be on the safe side and report them. When teachers have been given permission to report to the doctor directly, they will have access to the latest information regarding symptoms (teacher-doctor relating is discussed in Chapter 10).

Teachers also need to know when *not* to show concern. The coughing of a cystic fibrosis child is not contagious, and it is very important for him to cough in order to clear his lungs of mucus. The teacher must not try to get him to stop coughing. The child with juvenile rheumatoid arthritis takes high doses of aspirin, which causes buzzing in the ears. High tone hearing loss is concomitant. Also, if the aspirin is not taken at mealtime, or with milk, it can cause abdominal cramps. For the child with asthma, overuse of a broncho-dilator is dangerous. A child should not carry a broncho-dilator around with him but should use it only under supervision.[8] A teacher must insist that he be fully informed about the special aspects and requirements of a child's particular illness. He should not expect to know everything he needs to know without clear directives from the mother and the doctor.

Dealing with Emotionality

Psychological caretaking by the teacher will encompass giving comfort and reassurance to the child if he should become sick, have pain, or sustain a seizure in school. The class also must be reassured in such a circumstance. It is not the aim of this book to give instructions about handling medical emergencies, but the teacher should have information clearly in mind regarding how to proceed. Being gentle and safeguarding a child's self-esteem are the guiding principles of psychological caretaking.

Chronically ill children are frequently overly sensitive. They may burst into tears over a small rebuff, a mild criticism, or simply because they have made a mistake. Getting one spelling word wrong on a test or doing a page incorrectly because instructions have been misunderstood can open the floodgate, and tears begin to gush. This crying should not be thought of as babyish, immature, or as a serious emotional problem. It should be viewed simply as emotionality, and the child should be expected to recover quickly. Paying too much attention to sudden tears can make it worse, make the child overly self-conscious, and reinforce his sense of shame. Offer the child a tissue, put an arm or hand on his shoulder, reassure him that everyone makes mistakes, and tell him he'll soon be fine. If a few tears roll down the face, it is probably best to ignore them unless another child calls attention to them. In that case, say, "I think something has made Johnny feel bad." Then ask the child, who is probably feeling empathetic, if she would like to do something to comfort or reassure Johnny.

Appropriate Responses to the Seriously Ill Child

A seriously ill child wants and needs people near him and will attend school if at all possible. Yet he is likely to be apathetic and lethargic. He evokes sadness, sympathy, and anxiety in those around him. He does not seem to be himself or to react in expected ways. His lack of joy and lack of responsiveness make it difficult to relate to him. The teacher and the other children may feel uncertain about what to do or say. It is important to remember that the art of nonverbal communication is well developed in very young children. The very young have feelings to express before they have the words. Watch a two-year-old give a toy or some other treasured object to a crying child; a four-year-old bring his favorite blanket to his sad toddler sibling; a five-year-old offer a flower or card to a sick grandparent; a seven-year-old write a love note to an upset parent. In responding to a very ill child, adults and peers need to take their cues from these small, intuitive, compassionate creatures.

Picking up an ill child's dropped pencil; placing a box of tissues on his desk; offering a token of affection; taking her sweater from the back of her chair and placing it around her shoulders; opening a book to the right page; carrying a book without being asked to—these are all ways that teacher and classmates can show kindness and communicate caring. Without words, through actions, it is apparent that someone is noticing the ill child's state and anticipating his needs. If he looks cold, the sweater will bring warmth; if he has tears, it is all right, the tissues are there; if he lacks energy, picking up or carrying things for him will convey that this has been recognized. Offering a small token of affection, whether it is a piece of gum, a collecting item, or a note, will make an ill child feel accepted and cared about when his capacity to respond or reciprocate is limited.

Nonverbal communication puts less pressure on the one at the receiving end. It carries with it the idea that no response is expected. Of course, the receiver will most likely give a response, but it will be nonverbal also, and take little energy. Looking at the person making the gesture, or touching the object offered will be a response, low key though it is.

Some teachers are frightened at the prospect of having a chronically ill, or seriously ill, child in class. Their fear usually stems from lack of prior experience with such a child, or concern about the responsibility of handling a medical emergency. When parents, teacher, counselor, principal, and doctor assume conjoint responsibility, teachers can overcome their fears and will find that they have a lot to offer the chronically ill child. In the following three chapters, educators will learn how to help a child who has self-image problems, delayed emotional or social growth, or behavior problems.

NOTES

1. D. C. Klein and A. Ross, "Kindergarten Entry: A Study in Role Transition" in *Crisis Intervention, Selected Readings,* ed. H. J. Parad (New York: Family Service Association of America, 1965) pp. 145–146.

2. Roger Bibace and Mary E. Walsh, "Children's Conceptions of Illness" in *Children's Conceptions of Health, Illness, and Bodily Functions,* ed. R. Bibace and M. Walsh (San Francisco: Jossey-Bass, 1981) p. 36.

3. Joan Fassler, *Helping Children Cope: Mastering Stress through Books and Stories.* (New York: The Free Press, 1978) p. 27.

4. Edward H. Futterman and Irwin Hoffman, "Transient School Phobia in a Leukemic Child," *Journal of the American Academy of Child Psychiatry,* 9:477–493, 1970.

5. Paul Mussen and Nancy Eisenberg-Berg, *The Roots of Caring, Sharing, and Helping* (San Francisco: W. H. Freeman, 1977) pp. 74–100.

6. Patricia Greene, "The Child with Leukemia in the Classroom," *American Journal of Nursing,* 75:86–87, 1975.

7. Eugene E. Bleck and Donald A. Nagel, eds., *Physically Handicapped Children: A Medical Atlas for Teachers,* 2nd ed. (New York: Grune and Stratton, 1982) p. 427.

8. Bleck and Nagel, *Medical Atlas,* p. 40.

3

Coping with Changing Conditions: How Chronically Ill Children Differ from Handicapped Children

Cindy, a student in Mrs. Norbert's class, wears braces on her legs and uses a walker. Her legs were crushed in an automobile accident a year ago. Except for being crippled, she is healthy, bright, and normal. Kenneth, in Miss Bell's room, is confined to a wheelchair. He has spina bifida. Both are physically handicapped. What is the difference between them?

This chapter considers the features that distinguish the child with a chronic disorder from the handicapped and will show how a teacher can help a child who is distressed as a result of illness.

CHANGING NATURE OF HANDICAP IN CHRONIC ILLNESS

Whereas the children commonly considered handicapped (blind, deaf, retarded, psychotic, crippled) have permanent, generally unchanging conditions, chronically ill children have changing conditions. They get better and worse. They may be physically handicapped for a time and then okay; or the other way around, first physically okay, and later physically handicapped.

Cerebral Palsy and Spina Bifida

Children with cerebral palsy and spina bifida may begin life physically handicapped and get better function of their legs as a result of operations. The course of spina bifida is quite unpredictable, depending on the position of the neural tube defect, the nature of complications, and the outcome of operations. Some children may be ambulatory with braces, others wheelchair bound. The physical handicaps of children with cerebral palsy will either remain constant or get better, sometimes seeming to disappear. Fifty percent of children who are diagnosed as having cerebral palsy at age one no longer have neurological symptoms to substantiate such a diagnosis at age seven.[1]

Arthrogryposis and Osteogenesis Imperfecta

Arthrogryposis and osteogenesis imperfecta are other disorders that are evident at birth. A child with arthrogryposis may get better as a result of operations, but improved function is often only temporary. Children with osteogenesis imperfecta also may gain increasing mobility through operations with the use of braces. Occasionally, a child who has been wheelchair bound his whole life will be able to walk for the first time when he reaches adolescence.

Degenerative Disorders

For degenerative disorders such as Friedreich's ataxia and Duchenne muscular dystrophy, the process is the reverse. A physically perfect child gradually becomes more and more disabled. The child with muscular dystrophy may start needing help getting back to his feet from falling as early as four or five years of age. By ages seven to nine, he may need braces or a cane, and by ages eight to eleven he is usually confined to a wheelchair, with mechanical aids providing help to make his arms and hands still useful. Friedreich's ataxia has a more variable age of onset and a less predictable rate of progressive degeneration. Symptoms are occasionally evident in infancy, but more typically the diagnosis is not made until school age or adolescence.

Recurring Tumors

Children with recurring benign tumors will have no disability for a while and then become disabled in the part of the body where the tumors are growing. If they are growing in the mouth, the child will periodically lose the capacity to speak clearly. If they are on the hands, the ability to write and draw, and feed and dress oneself may become limited. If they are on the feet, the child may have to use crutches for a while. These children undergo repeated operations for the removal of the tumors.

Scoliosis

Scoliosis is a late-developing physical disability, with onset usually in late childhood or early adolescence. A girl, just as she is becoming concerned about being attractive and feminine, must suddenly start wearing a brace. When all other measures do not stop the progression of the spine curvature, surgery and many months in a body cast may be necessary.

Later onset of physical handicap also occurs where a specific disease process has caused joint deformity. Joint damage may result from juvenile rheumatoid arthritis as well as from hemophilia.

INVISIBLE HANDICAPS

Children who are physically handicapped, but not visibly so, are those whose chronic illness places severe restrictions on their physical activity. Severe lung disorders, such as cystic fibrosis and asthma, juvenile rheumatoid arthritis, kidney disorders, heart conditions, and sickle cell anemia, are examples of invisible physical handicaps. The arthritic child needs to exercise her joints regularly but must avoid twisting movements and overstressing the joints. Children with lung disorders must not have strenuous exercise. The same is true of many children who have heart conditions. For most, physical activity must be continually monitored in terms of the kind, duration, and climatic conditions under which it takes place. This requires regular vigilance on the part of the supervising adult, and appropriate respect for his disorder on the part of the child. Because sports, particularly for boys, are a big part of life during late childhood and adolescence, an asthmatic boy might disregard his restrictions and put himself at risk for more flare-ups of his illness. On the other hand, for the hemophilic boy, participation in most sports is beneficial. Because joint bleeding is capricious, not necessarily brought on by bumps and falls, moderate exercise that allows the boy to feel as normal as possible is usually suggested by his doctor.

OTHER WAYS IN WHICH THE CHRONICALLY ILL AND THE HANDICAPPED DIFFER

There are several features that distinguish chronic disorders from handicaps. The most dramatic of these is that chronic illnesses are often life-threatening or life-limiting. For certain illnesses, early diagnosis and treatment may be of life-and-death importance. For other illnesses, such as epilepsy, asthma, juvenile diabetes mellitus, and hemophilia, the death rate is low, but the symptoms can require emergency treatment. The symptoms may be very frightening, making it look as if the child could die. Childhood cancer, until recently a fatal disease, is now considered a life-threatening illness. At least 50 percent of children with cancer survive.[2] Cystic fibrosis, Duchenne muscular dystrophy, Friedreich's ataxia, and some of the kidney, heart, and blood disorders, are life-limiting. Death will usually come in adolescence or early adulthood unless complications cause an earlier death. Improved treatments have greatly reduced the morbidity and mortality of many illnesses, but no way has yet been found to stop the progression of degenerative disorders. Prevention of inheritable disorders through genetic counseling and family planning must suffice to reduce the tragedy of progressive disorders, until other approaches can offer some hope.

Somewhat different from the life-threatening aspect, but similar in its impact, is the fact that chronic illnesses are rarely cured. There is an uneven course with most illnesses, but a lifetime vulnerability is the norm. About 60 to 70 percent of children with juvenile rheumatoid arthritis are free of the disease within ten years of onset but can still develop the adult form of the disease.[3] Asthma is another illness that generally improves with age, but one is never free of it. Capricious diseases, such as juvenile diabetes mellitus and hemophilia, which have periods of exacerbation with no known cause, often settle down to a relative calm by midadolescence.

The changeable course of an illness, the unpredictable future outcome, and, in many instances, the suffering of chronic pain, are features that distinguish the chronically ill from the handicapped. Also, most children with chronic disorders experience hospitalization; many undergo surgery. Growth failure is a consequence for some chronically ill children. Incurring infections is often hazardous, and the danger of complications a continuing worry. Fears, both anticipatory to what they must undergo (surgeries, tests, and so on) and as a result of hospitalization, surgery, and the bodily experience of the illness, are common.

Pain

Handicapped children are no more subject to pain than are normal children. However, pain is part of the experience of chronic illness, although it may be much less for children with certain disorders than for others. Since pain is invisible, others are not always aware that a child is in pain. Children with juvenile rheumatoid arthritis often complain that no one seems to appreciate or understand that they have pain.[4] Pain for the hemophiliac is the danger alert that a bleeding episode has started. Pain may be the main symptom of an attack of the illness, as in migraine or abdominal seizure equivalents, or it may be an early signal that trouble is brewing and they need to see their doctor. When a child has a known chronic illness, a teacher must give serious attention to the child's reports of pain.

Children with sickle cell anemia are in excruciating pain during a sickling crisis. They may require narcotic medications. The child with juvenile rheumatoid arthritis probably has the most continual pain. These children's joints must be kept mobile; when the joints are stiff, the exercises needed to make them move can be very painful.

Young children have difficulty comprehending pain. They usually think their pain and suffering is punishment for some wrongdoing. Older children may resent having pain and are prone to blame their parents for it. They feel angry that they must endure the pain. They expect parents and doctors to be able to make the pain go away and become disagreeable with them when they can't.[5]

Teachers cannot make pain go away and should not offer too much sympathy. After comfort has been offered, a child should be expected to do what his doctor says he should do. Children who view their pain as a challenge will learn to tolerate it better. Focusing on the sensation of pain itself can cause the pain to seem more intense. Therefore, these children need to become so engrossed in a learning project that they can become distracted from their pain.

Effects on Growth

Disorders of physical growth and development are common in children with sickle cell disease, cystic fibrosis, juvenile rheumatoid arthritis, heart disease, and chronic kidney disease. Long-term steroid treatment causes short stature as well as a puffy, round face. When growth has been delayed because of drug treatments, there is usually catch-up growth after the medication has been stopped. Some catch-up growth may occur after surgical repair of a congenital heart condition, but the child doesn't usually achieve normal growth potential.[6]

Children who are very small for their age are commonly perceived as much younger than they actually are. Age mates may exclude them because of this. Boys in particular can be extremely sensitive about their small size. The way this sensitivity is handled has an impact on personality development. It is important that a teacher discourage other children from teasing an ill child about his size. If his growth failure is the result of medication, he can be reminded that he will eventually catch up when he no longer has to take the medication. The teacher should consult the doctor before offering this kind of reassurance. Handicapped children do not generally experience similar growth problems.

Complications

The treatments that remedy or control their conditions may pose a hazard for chronically ill children. Chemotherapeutic agents lower resistance and make a child susceptible to infections. The disease-fighting mechanisms may also be rendered ineffective by the primary illness or the effect of treatments, and the relentless occurrence of infection can become extremely dangerous to health. In fact, death may be caused by a secondary infection rather than by the primary illness.

There are other consequences of the necessary medical treatments that create serious complications. Diabetics are vulnerable to insulin reactions and must be given glucose immediately to prevent a medical crisis. Children who receive many blood transfusions may contract hepatitis. Medications used to control seizures may affect the liver as well as the red and white blood cells. Anticonvulsant medicines may also alter mental processing functions or cause behavioral or personality changes. Cognitive impairment may occur as a consequence of the drugs and radiation used to treat cancer. One study showed neurological difficulties in 50 percent of a small group of leukemic children treated.[7]

There are a variety of complications that occur with spina bifida. Hydrocephalus, requiring shunting, occurs in many when the neural tube defect is closed at birth. The shunt itself may cause difficulties over time, requiring correction. Urinary tract infections and kidney problems are prevalent. Neurosurgery and orthopedic surgery are common.

The complications of serious kidney disease include high blood pressure and anemia. Children with juvenile rheumatoid arthritis (oligoarticular type) may develop inflammation in their eyes, which can lead to blindness if not treated promptly.

Overall, the danger of complications poses a significant threat to the chronically ill child. Chronic anxiety for the parent and child is a concomitant of this threat. Unwarranted reassurance should not be extended in an effort to reduce anxiety, although supporting the hopes of parent and child is always appropriate.

Fears

The chronically ill child has many sources of fear: fear of needles; fear of the effect of medicines, surgery, and treatments; fear of hospitalization; fear of bodily mutilation; and the worst fear of all—the possibility of death.

All school-age children (normal and handicapped) typically have fears of bodily harm because they have become aware of the many sources of external threat. These fears will be greatly exaggerated for the chronically ill child because of additional fears stemming from his illness and what he has experienced as a result of it. Children with convulsive disorders fear loss of consciousness and strange behavior because these things happen to them when they have seizures. Such children may need to control others, or have control of a situation; that is, control issues may be overly important to them. They may become anxious and frightened if another child loses his self-control or starts acting strangely.

Children with respiratory illness (asthma, cystic fibrosis) commonly harbor fears of suffocating, drowning, or dying while asleep. Children with bleeding disorders, such as hemophilia, are often afraid they will bleed to death.[8] Children sometimes conceal their fears in their efforts to be brave and show courage. These children often have bad dreams and nightmares. Their fears are expressed in their sleep. Adults are often unaware that these children have such intense underlying fears unless they guess it from the dreams that are reported.

When a child sees how frightened and upset adults become when she starts having symptoms, she will become frightened also. The very young child does not yet have sufficient knowledge to consciously fear (that is, anticipate) bodily damage and death, but she can assimilate fear by identification. Older children also assimilate the anxiety and worry of their parents. With more developed cognitive abilities, however, they can understand what is happening and respond more quickly to verbal reassurance offered by the medical staff. Although many children learn to hide their fears of bodily harm while learning to master them, some chronically ill children sense that they must be protected from harm and that openly expressing their fears will help to keep them safe. The teacher should not be surprised if a child who has a known medical problem expresses a lot of worries about his body.

She should offer reassurance if she is sure about her predictions, show concern about symptoms when appropriate, and help the child learn to differentiate between significant and insignificant symptoms. This requires accurate knowledge of the illness, which all teachers (as well as principals) should have.

CHILDREN'S COPING MECHANISMS

It is important to recognize children's coping mechanisms because teachers and parents need to encourage and support the effort a child makes to cope. Although all children, normal and handicapped, have fears, conflicts, and anger to come to terms with as they grow, chronically ill children have additional ones arising out of their illness, medical treatments, and hospitalizations.

Children have a limited range of coping mechanisms, but these expand as their cognitive abilities and academic skills develop. Pretend play is a young child's mode for confronting fears, anger, and conflicts. In the natural course of events, a child's wishes and impulses may collide with those of caretaking adults and peers. The child may then turn to a favorite stuffed animal or doll and work out her mixed feelings through talk and play. The child becomes the authoritarian adult, denies her doll's "wish" and then comforts it. The doll may "fight back" in protest, using all the persuasive tactics it knows, and the child, role-playing the parent, will give in. In one way or another, the child either pretends she has gotten her wish, or knows she is loved and feels comforted even if she hasn't gotten her wish.

This mechanism of pretend play is also used to deal with fears and to overcome distress. It is the young child's way of assimilating new learning. It is her emotional safety valve and the organizer of her emerging intellect. Parents and teachers must nurture the child's role-playing talents, encourage this form of play, and be accepting of the ideas, feelings, and solutions she projects in her play.

After a dreaded hospitalization during which a child has experienced many indignities that violate his sense of privacy regarding his body, invasive procedures, pain, and possibly restraint, his rage may be great. He may be able to get over his rage if he can do all those awful things to his favorite stuffed animal, a doll, or puppet.[9] Then, role-playing the child puppet's encounter with the doctor or nurse puppet, he may have the child puppet scream and protest that it will not have the medicine or procedure. When he does this, he is acting out feelings that he could not express in the real situation.

Magical thinking, the characteristic mode of thought of very young children, is another useful mechanism for dealing with fears, anger, and distress. Eerie machines can be transformed into benign and friendly objects through magical thinking. One can believe that an absent parent can be made to appear by the fairy godmother. When the child invents magic words and pretends that some object is the magic lamp or magic wand, he can become the friendly magician or fairy godmother and set things right for the hurt and upset child that he is.

These mechanisms of pretend play and magical solutions are gradually replaced in school-age children with new forms, made possible by their increasing skills and abilities. However, some older children continue to utilize pretend play and magical thinking because they are such effective coping tools. Adults may be tempted to discourage pretend play in the older child, who has reached the level of logical thought. However, many ill and emotionally disturbed children still need to make use of these forms, and they should be allowed to do so.

Older children, with more advanced mental development, and having developed the skills of reading, writing, and drawing, will have new modes for dealing with emotional tensions. These older children can identify with characters in stories and movies. They can release emotions through reading and writing poetry, writing creative stories, and drawing pictures. They can act in a play, become another person for a moment. They can make up jokes and get involved in funny stories and movies that make them laugh. Their developing sense of humor will be a helpful tool for overcoming painful thoughts and feelings.

Older children can also use knowledge as a coping mechanism. By learning to understand her illness and how to care for herself, an older child can become competent in handling potential emergencies. This will make her feel less anxious. She can be taught how to deal with the curiosity of other children. She can understand why she has certain restrictions. Knowledge can lead to self-acceptance and reduction of anger and fear.

HELPING AN ANXIOUS CHILD

Unlike the unchanging, permanent condition of the handicapped child, the uncertain, unpredictable course of illness makes the chronically ill child prone to constant or recurring anxiety. Anxiety may stem from fears or from his responsibility for keeping himself safe. The school-age child begins to realize that he shares in the responsibility for keeping himself safe. He knows that an episode of his illness must receive prompt medical attention when it starts. He must learn to know the symptoms and to recognize the signs that indicate he needs medical help. There is no way to predict when an episode will happen. A certain amount of a child's energy will be consumed in anxious anticipation or worry about becoming ill without warning. He may report many minor insignificant somatic symptoms because he is fearful that he may become critically ill or that he will not get medical help in time. He may fear going on field trips because he will be out of touch with his usual support system.

An anxious child in the classroom may move about a lot, have great difficulty settling down to work, and be unable to concentrate for very long periods. The teacher should recognize that this restless behavior very likely reflects the child's anxiety. Even if the activity level is of such a degree to be labeled hyperactive, it is most probably the result of anxiety. The side effects of some medications can make a child hyperactive, so this possibility must be investigated first. Then, rather than focusing on the child's activity level as such, as something that must be corrected, the teacher should consider how best to keep the child on task and lengthen his span of concentration.

The Buddy System

Assigning an anxious child a working mate is a good way to start. The child picked to be the work buddy should be a conscientious worker and a person who has easy rapport with peers. This does not mean she has to be one of the top students, as her job will be to keep the anxious child in his seat and working, not to perform as a peer tutor. It is possible that the work buddy needs no further instruction than to have her job defined for her. However, if she seems uncertain, the teacher should give her specific things to do: "If John loses his place, tell him where we are working; if John starts to get up, tap his arm gently and ask him if he has finished the first task (set of problems, written exercise, or whatever). Show John how far you have gotten and see if he is there yet, or if he can catch up with you," and so on.

The buddy system is the method of choice for children of second grade or higher. Immaturity factors may make it ineffective for first graders and for some second graders. For children under seven (and some seven-year-olds), placing the child in a seat near the teacher and using personal gestures (smiles, pats on the arm or back, looking at his work often) and concrete rewards (stars, stickers of any kind, a special play time) will probably be necessary.

Counseling

In order to get at the source of the child's anxiety, the school counselor should meet with him individually, on a weekly basis. Also, peer counseling groups with other chronically ill children as participants are often available through a local hospital or within the community.

If a child becomes acutely anxious about being in school (or going on a field trip) because he fears he will not get medical help in time if he needs it, he should be reassured in concrete ways. If his fears are out of proportion to the known facts of his illness, the teacher should first make sure she has correct information about his illness. A phone discussion with the parent or doctor is indicated. She then should show the child that she has emergency phone numbers and, when necessary, things that will be needed in an emergency. If his worry is about a field trip, tell him that the bus can be stopped in order to call the doctor, or that the bus driver can change the route and drive directly to the nearest hospital. Tell him the names and addresses of the hospitals that are in the vicinity of where the bus will be going. Let him write these down if he wants to. Most likely, nothing serious will happen on the trip, but the child is showing a sense of responsibility when he expresses these anxious concerns.

When ill children become so anxious about their bodies and what will happen to them that their minds are full of catastrophic thoughts and fantasies, it is very difficult to get them interested in the ordinary tasks of a school day. However, the teacher is obligated to try.

MODIFYING THE CURRICULUM

The need to make changes in the curriculum is indicated when a child does not respond to regular school tasks. Such a child may be daydreaming to escape from the realities of her illness or from her anxious concerns about herself, her family, or her future. Teachers usually feel frustrated in their efforts to motivate a turned-off child to do work, not realizing that an alternate approach might prove successful. I believe a teacher should feel successful if he is able to engage such a child in *any* kind of academic work. In the following section, I will discuss one approach that is possible. Once a teacher begins to think in terms of curriculum modification, changing the task rather than continuing to look for ways to get the child to do the regular tasks, other ideas will probably come to mind. A second purpose of curriculum modification is to increase the quality of life for children with progressive disorders, shortened life spans, and for those who are terminally ill.

Getting a Child Absorbed in Learning

Special fears or preoccupations often cause a chronically ill child to be inattentive or unresponsive in school. If he becomes involved in a learning project, he can perhaps forget his self-concerns. In order to divert such a child from pain, fears, or worries, the task must really grab his interest. Other factors that will enhance his ability to become absorbed will be working together with another student and having activity as an aspect of the project. Perhaps it would also help if he could receive recognition by sharing the outcome of the project with others—his own class or other classes. It is important to let such a child develop the idea for the project himself. It may be a project outside of the regular curriculum, centering around a personal interest or some area of special ability. Once he has chosen his project, he should be permitted to pick a classmate to participate with him. The teacher should make suggestions, but should not force ideas upon him. If the ill child does not want a partner in his project, he should not be required to have one. Perhaps he would rather involve a parent or a sibling in the project.

If a child is so deeply absorbed that he cannot participate in a teacher's efforts to get him involved in a special project, a more creative approach is needed.

The following story about Jimmy shows another direction that a teacher can take with a preoccupied child who is turned off to learning. Jimmy was enrolled in a special class, but even there he was "doing nothing" while in school. He was relatively noncommunicative and spent his time wandering around, crawling under desks, or fiddling with small objects brought from home.

Jimmy, age ten and a half, was born with a stricture of his esophagus that had caused repeated medical crises throughout his short life. His esophagus had to be stretched periodically during infancy and his early years. Emergencies were caused when a piece of food would become caught in his esophagus. When referred for psychological evaluation, Jimmy was asked to make some drawings. His pictures indicated that he was acutely aware of the financial burden his condition had caused and also of the severe anxiety that pervaded the family. (The family had organized itself around Jimmy's disorder. His father carried with him to each new evaluation a three-inch thick notebook containing reports of all that had been done for Jimmy.) When asked to draw a person, Jimmy drew a robber with a huge bag of money in each hand. He represented his esophageal stricture by a heavily emphasized zipper. He said that this person was a man who had just robbed a bank. His family drawing depicted all the family members working on a wrecked car. The extremely heavy shading reflected the intensity of the family anxiety, as well as his own.

Although Jimmy's performance on tests showed he was below average, his drawings contained many abstract symbols reflecting above-average intellectual potential. In representing his esophagus as a zipper, he seemed to be projecting a fantasized solution to his problem (that is, if food got caught he could open the zipper to let it pass.) The robber probably symbolized several concerns. Jimmy felt that he had robbed the family because his medical condition placed a severe strain on its finances. The idea of robbing a bank reflected a wish to find a solution to those financial problems. He was also perhaps making a statement that he felt robbed of his normalcy.

In his family drawing, the wrecked car represented both his own condition and that of the family. The fact that everyone in the picture was working hard to keep the car going correctly symbolized Jimmy's perceptions that the family was pulling together; but both he and his family were extremely vulnerable to becoming disabled—breaking down. In the drawing, he placed himself under the car. He seemed to be projecting the idea that if the car (family) broke down, he would be dead (crushed by the car, not gotten to the hospital in time).

The remarkable thing was that Jimmy had sustained his concentration, while making the drawings, for a very long period of time. He was obviously capable of paying attention and of concentration, although it took something of significance for him to show it. The ideas, feelings, and fantasies that formed the basis of his pictorial symbols were of sufficient importance to him to sustain his concentration and attention.

Jimmy's teacher needed to find something of an academic nature that would be as engrossing for him as the picture drawing had been. What clues did the drawings offer that might be a starting point? The most obvious one was that Jimmy drew well and liked to draw. Making drawings to illustrate his written work or what he had read or observed would be an important activity for him. There were two major symbols in his drawings: the bank robber and the wrecked car needing repair.

One of Jimmy's preoccupations had to do with money as a way to solve the family's problems. A unit on banking, with a banker's concerns about getting robbed as a secondary theme, would seem an enticing possibility as something to grab Jimmy's interest and one that could involve the whole class. Such a unit could incorporate math, economics, social studies, and even history (the history of money, banking, or both). Making loans to people who had big medical bills would be a significant aspect of the thinking and planning. Language arts could be brought in through the activity of constructing and acting out a play about a robber who was really a good person, such as Robin Hood, who stole money to help people. Constructing and setting up a bank, making the play money, and organizing how the bank would operate and do business would be the more enjoyable aspects of the unit and would provide an excellent opportunity to practice organizing skills.

The symbol of the wrecked car offered a possibility for an individual learning unit. Thinking and reading about repairing cars would seem to fit into Jimmy's symbolic system. The teacher might begin by having Jimmy list all the internal parts of a car that he knew could cause disablement of the whole car. He could be asked to write everything he knew about keeping cars in good repair, how much parts and labor would cost, and so on. Once Jimmy was sufficiently absorbed by the subject, the teacher could direct him to appropriate reading material. The study of repairing cars could be expanded, as Jimmy was able to get more involved in learning, to studying the history of the auto industry or to categorizing types and uses of cars. The wide variety of uses of cars and other motor vehicles could lead the student in any of a variety of directions. In this way, the original topic would serve to seed many other interests and create the momentum needed to get a child to stop thinking only about himself and his family's problems.

There are many preoccupied children other than those who are chronically ill sitting in every classroom. The teacher who learns the skill of taking cues from a child's drawings to stimulate his interest in academic activities will find wide application for it. If a child is able to transform his emotional dilemmas into graphic symbols (pictures) as Jimmy did, the teacher should feel challenged to get him to transform them into written symbols (stories), information gathering, thinking, and calculating as well. Even children who do not draw well are usually so eager to express themselves in some form that they readily draw pictures when asked.

If a child like Jimmy is sitting in a regular classroom doing nothing, the teacher could ask him to draw some action pictures about anything he wants to draw. Maybe he has a story in his head that he wants to tell in picture form. The teacher then should find a private time to talk to the child about the pictures. She should ask, "What's this?" "What's happening here?" and any other questions suggested by what the child has put in the drawing. The idea is to get at the meanings of the objects and actions and see if the child will weave them into a story. If a story emerges, the teacher can then ask, "How does it turn out?" The teacher may wish to share her thoughts about the child's picture symbols with other teachers or special staff to get their ideas or additional feedback before developing an academic project for the child based on clues in his pictures.

One common pictorial symbol used by children deserves special mention because it can be misunderstood. Many children—particularly boys—who are in severe conflict or who feel threatened or scared seem to draw nothing but war pictures. This does not reflect a violent nature in the child, but rather his sense of impending catastrophe, his sense of vulnerability. Tapping into the underlying emotional dilemma is an important aspect of converting a child's graphic symbols into academic interests. One ten-year-old boy obsessed by potential catastrophe knew a lot about every catastrophic global event of the past six months. These ranged from tidal waves to forest fires, from volcanic eruptions to hurricanes, and included events such as a plane crash and a ship that sank. The point is that in these instances, it is catastrophe— not the concrete features of a picture story—that is the clue to be used. In reading or writing about how catastrophes can be prevented, the child makes progress in mastering conflicts and fears.

Considering the Quality of Life

Curriculum modifications that provide maximum satisfaction and minimum displeasure are particularly important for chronically ill children. These children have experienced much discouragement, boredom, and discomfort in the process of their medical treatment. They are in great need of having a rewarding school experience. They may have developed habits of daydreaming to distract themselves from feeling miserable or bored when their illness confined them. They may, more easily than other children, become discouraged or distracted if they are required to work endlessly on something that is too difficult, tedious, or unrewarding.

Consideration of the quality of life may stimulate thinking about curriculum modifications even more for children with degenerative disorders, those who have only a short time to live, and for children who have a shortened life span (expected to live only until early adulthood). An emphasis on academic skill development may not be the most important thing the school has to offer these children. Staying in classes with friends, having a chance to spend more time on the arts, or developing a special skill or new interest may be of greater importance.

In making the decision to modify the curriculum for a child with a shortened life span it is wise to consider how a less well-liked subject, such as math, can be combined with a high-interest subject, such as history. Math would not really be ignored, it would just be an aspect of the more important (to the child) study of history. For example, in studying the westward movement in American history, calculating total distances by adding the distance between stops, time/distance ratios, amounts of various kinds of supplies needed, costs, and so on, would constitute the child's math curriculum. Writing a journal about events that must be anticipated and how to handle them would be an aspect of language arts that could be incorporated in the study. Thus, no part of the regular curriculum would be left out, but the emphasis would be on learning something historical.

Improving an ill child's quality of life may mean reducing assignments that are tedious (writing is tedious for the child with muscular dystrophy or cerebral palsy) and increasing his exposure to subject matter that nourishes him (reading an exciting adventure story). It may also mean allowing him to stay with his peers even when his academic skills are well below those of his classmates. It does not make sense to require a twelve-year-old boy with muscular dystrophy to remain in sixth grade when all his friends are going on to junior high school, even though his skills are only at fifth grade level. In other instances, providing a very ill child with the haven of a special class may be the alternative needed to improve his quality of life.

Concerning Parents

Parents should not be asked whether they want the school to make quality-of-life modifications for a child. The reason is that parents do not want to focus on the imminence of the terminal phase of their child's illness. They have very likely decided that their child should lead a normal life as long as possible. Changes in the curriculum or in expectations connote something other than normalcy. Teachers should intuitively make changes. Parents will be pleased if their child is happy. They are not going to be aware that anything special has been done for their child, and no one should try to make them aware of this.

All teachers do not have the same degree of confidence about attempting new curriculum ideas. This may reflect either a lack of experience or a previous experience of having been criticized for being innovative. It is always wise to discuss curriculum changes for special children with the principal before implementing them. If a principal is extremely conservative, she may not encourage the type of creative approaches I have suggested. However, such a principal may become more liberal if a teacher dares to try new ideas and demonstrates that they work.

NOTES

1. Karin B. Nelson and Jonas H. Ellenberg, "Children Who Outgrew Cerebral Palsy." *Pediatrics,* Vol. 69, 5:529–535, May 1982, p. 534.

2. Gerald P. Koocher and John E. O'Malley, *The Damocles Syndrome: Psychosocial Consequences of Surviving Childhood Cancer.* (New York: McGraw-Hill, 1981) pp. 1 and 33.

3. Eugene E. Bleck and Donald A. Nagel, eds., *Physically Handicapped Children: A Medical Atlas for Teachers* 2nd ed. (NY: Grune and Stratton, 1982) p. 423.

4. Bleck and Nagel, *Medical Atlas,* p. 429.

5. Ake Mattson, "Long-term Physical Illness in Childhood: A Challenge to Psychosocial Adaptation." *Pediatrics,* 50:801, 1972, p. 803.

6. Bleck and Nagel, *Medical Atlas,* p. 461.

7. Sue McIntosh and others, "Chronic Neurological Disturbance in Childhood Leukemia." *Cancer,* 37:853–857, 1976.

8. Mattson, "Long-Term Physical Illness," p. 804.

9. Mary Ann Adams, "A Hospital Play Program, Helping Children with Serious Illness." *American Journal of Orthopsychiatry,* 46 (3): 416, 1976, p. 421.

4

How Teachers Can Help an Ill Child Cope, Socialize, and Build Self-Esteem

Juanita was aware that kids kept their distance from her. She thought it was because of the scars on her leg and the funny way she walked. Her mother disagreed. "It's because we are Mexican," she told Juanita. "It takes time for our people to be accepted here. The boys and girls will be more friendly if you show how polite and kind you are." Juanita kept her scars covered and managed to make friends after a while. Now, at age twelve, she was in a new school, and the kids turned away from her no matter how friendly and nice she was. "Mother was wrong," she told herself. "It *is* because of my scars and limp that kids don't like me."

FEELING DIFFERENT: CHRONIC ILLNESS AFFECTS SELF-ESTEEM

Chronically ill children have problems feeling okay about themselves and have problems with socialization. The teacher has a significant role in helping them with building self-esteem and gaining acceptance.

All children who have physical disorders feel different, whether or not others see their difference. What makes them feel this way? Is it the frequent need for medical tests? the many trips to doctor or hospital? the daily requirements to take pills, be given shots, or do exercises? the fright aroused in others when they start to wheeze or have seizures? or the specific sense that some parts of their bodies do not function properly? Regardless of whether adults wish to think they are normal, chronically ill children, even those with a very mild disorder, are going to feel that they are not normal to some extent.

This feeling is not always expressed directly by a child. Perhaps young children do not know how to ask questions about what is happening to their bodies. Perhaps they intuitively know that it would make their parents anxious and uncomfortable if they were to ask.

The Epileptic Child

The following story about Rosalie illustrates the ways she experienced being different. Although she has normal intelligence, the nature of her illness was never discussed with her. The drawings she made conveyed her need for information, which she was too inhibited to ask for in words.

Rosalie is a seven-year-old whose epilepsy was diagnosed at age three, shortly after her younger sister was born. For years, she has had to go to the hospital at regular intervals for blood tests to determine the level of the anticonvulsant medicine in her body. When she has a convulsion, she doesn't know what has happened to her, why she is sleepy in the middle of the day, and why everyone is hovering over her, asking if she is all right. With a new baby to take care of, as well as a three-year-old to give medicine to regularly and take to the doctor often, Rosalie's mother found it easier to keep on bathing, dressing, and feeding Rosalie, rather than training and encouraging her to do these things for herself. When Marie, the younger sister, was old enough to begin to dress and bathe herself, she took to it happily. However, Rosalie, having been waited on for years, was now extremely dependent. Rosalie dawdled and played until her mother did everything for her. In school, she also dawdled, but no one would take her coat off for her, and she was always late getting to her seat. The children stared, and the teacher acted angry. Rosalie could see that she was different because her mother dressed her, but not her younger sister. She was also treated differently by others at school. The teacher always insisted that someone go with her to the bathroom (the nurse thought this was wise) while other children could go alone. She knew that her body did peculiar things that she had no control over. She had to go for blood tests and take medicine all the time, something Marie didn't have to do.

Rosalie conveyed her sense of being different by drawing a picture of a person with two sets of eyes, two sets of ears, and two mouths, when the psychologist asked her to draw a person. She most likely *felt* as if she had two mouths and two sets of eyes and ears because at times her eyes, ears, and mouth did peculiar things. At other times, they acted normal. She did not know what caused her head and body to do those things. No one had ever talked to her about her epilepsy. By drawing the picture, she conveyed her need for information as well as her inner sense of being different.

CHANGE IN SELF-IMAGE

A child's self-image changes during the process of her adaptation to her disorder. Even if there are no external changes in the body, a child can have an internalized sense that her body is damaged. She thinks "there is something wrong with me; I'm not all right." The very existence of the illness can make her think and feel this way. She has experienced the medical treatments and the changes in her body's reactions, and she knows that her body is not totally okay. Rosalie has an inner sense that something is wrong with her. She can't see what makes her different, but she experiences it.

The Child with Skin Disorders

Henry is a boy who can see his body changing. Here is what happened to him.

At the age of eight, Henry developed a skin disorder that caused him to lose the pigment in his skin. The blotches started in a small way, but continued to spread. By the age of ten, he had brown and white blotches all over his arms, legs, and body. He thought he looked like a giraffe and was very concerned that his face would become blotchy. He thought that his disorder was some kind of cancer, and he didn't know why this had happened to him. He didn't know whether it had serious consequences for his future. His doctor had told him nothing except that there was no treatment for his condition. At the moment, the process of change in coloration of his skin had stopped, but he dreaded the possibility that it would start again. He occasionally thought that others were afraid of him, that maybe he was like a leper. He kept his arms and legs covered and wore long-sleeved shirts and long pants, even in hot weather, because he sensed that everyone stared at him when his arms and legs were exposed.

CHILDREN NEED INFORMATION

Both Rosalie and Henry were in need of information about what was happening to their bodies. They both felt they couldn't ask. Although the doctor should explain the illness or condition to the child, there are many doctors who do not do this. Teachers should ask parents if anyone has talked to the child about his illness. Children will not ask questions unless there is an atmosphere of openness. Adults must initiate the process of giving ill children information about themselves.

A change in self-image can make a child quite self-conscious and aware of his wounds and scars, from needles, operations, or treatments, even when these are not observable by others. If a child approaches others by directing attention to his scars or deformities or by announcing himself as a child who has asthma, diabetes, arthritis, or cancer, he will be communicating his intense awareness of being different.

The Teacher's Response

The teacher or other adult should not interpret this kind of behavior as a bid for pity or special privilege. It is a child's way of letting others know that he is anxious about himself, that he is not sure he can meet normal expectations, and that he has had experiences that are different from those of other children. He is saying, in essence, that he is in need of special understanding.

The teacher must respond to the child who calls blatant attention to his illness by effecting a matter-of-fact manner, showing an interest in the scars or crippling, and asking what it means to have the particular illness that the child identifies. For example, when she says, "I am a diabetic," she can be told, "Tell me what that means." She should not be ashamed or criticized for approaching others in this manner, but she can be taught more subtle ways to share her anxieties with others.

The Child with Tumors

Ernest is a boy who succeeded in frightening the whole class because he did not know how to handle his worries about himself.

> Ernest, age nine, was anxious about his body because of recurring tumors on his hands, arms, and legs. These tumors required periodic surgical removal. The most recent tumor appeared near his temple. This brought Ernest to a state of near panic, as he was sure the tumor would affect his brain. He began to express his fears openly to other children, displaying the bumps and scars on his body and telling the others he would probably die.
>
> The teacher noticed that anxiety was spreading among the other children in the class, who were worried about Ernest's

mysterious malady. They feared for his life; they wondered if such a thing could happen to them.

After consultation with Ernest's parents and the school counselor, it was agreed that two things must be done: The class must be reassured and freed from their anxious concern and Ernest must learn to deal with his anxieties in a way that would not frighten and upset others. Ernest's teacher, his counselor, and his mother worked together on a project to reassure the class. Ernest's mother told the class what was known about the disorder and assured them that it would not happen to them. It was not known when and where the tumors would occur, but the doctors thought it highly unlikely that the brain would become involved. Ernest did not have cancer. The disorder was not catching.

The students in the class were asked to write Ernest a note expressing their feelings about his condition. They were to write any ideas they could think of that might help Ernest worry less about himself. The counselor began to see Ernest weekly to give him the opportunity to confront his fears, play out his catastrophic expectations, and find ways to share his fears with others without creating undue alarm in them.

PARENTAL LACK OF AWARENESS OF THE CHILD'S FEARS, WORRIES, ANXIETIES

Most parents are realistically concerned about their child's chronic illness. Some are overconcerned; they tend to hover, notice small changes in a child's appearance, and be oversolicitous. However, some families minimize or ignore the child's illness. These parents want their child to feel 100 percent normal. They think it is best to forget about the illness, believing that the child will be fine as long as he takes his medicine, shots, or whatever.

A chronically ill child in such a family cannot share his fears and worries. It surprises the parents to learn that their child feels insecure and uncertain about whether his parents will be appropriately protective of him. Children with mild forms of juvenile rheumatoid arthritis or asthma are sometimes more prone to develop emotional problems than are children who have a more severe form of the disease. This is primarily because their families seem to forget that they have a chronic illness except when they have symptoms.[1] Such children may pretend to have symptoms to convey to parents or teachers that they are worried about themselves. Danny was such a boy.

Danny was a six-year-old boy who had had asthma as a young child but had been free of symptoms and attacks for two years. His mother claimed that he was well. She admired his seemingly high intellectual capabilities and had great expectations for him. In school, he acted incompetent, performed poorly, and did not socialize with the other children. One day in class, he started to pant and said, "I think I'm having an asthmatic attack." The teacher intuitively knew he was not having an attack and told him so. She explained to him that it was very important not to pretend about such a serious thing, but she did not know why he did it. When he was referred for psychological evaluation, it was found that he had a great deal of body anxiety and was not feeling protected and nurtured. He was rebelling in school by acting incompetent (he was actually bright and learning satisfactorily) because of his mother's excessive intellectual expectations and her nonchalant attitude about his body concerns and his illness.

SENSE OF ISOLATION

Chronically ill children are literally isolated from siblings, classmates, and familiar adults when they are confined in the hospital. Because their experiences are so different and they cannot participate in many of the normal activities of siblings and peers, they begin to feel that they have nothing in common with other children. For example, leaving a group to receive medical attention, to take a pill, or to get a shot adds to their sense of isolation. Eating a special diet makes a child stand out from others, isolates him as one who is not doing as others do.

Chronically ill children are going to feel isolated for one reason or another, no matter what. However, the degree and intensity of this feeling can be kept at a tolerable level if adults are aware and help ill children feel included whenever possible. Child peers can be instructed to say, for example: "That's okay, we'll wait" or "We'll still be here" when the child has to leave a group for some medical reason. The teacher also gets this idea across when she speaks for the children, "I'm sure the group will wait for you."

STRESS SAMENESS OF FEELINGS AND DESIRES

Although most chronically ill children will have a sense of being different, they must come to realize that their being different is only a small part of their total self. Adults need to be careful not to reinforce feelings of differentness. Teacher (and parent) should challenge the child's sense of being different by emphasizing that she is more like everyone else than she is different. In doing this, the teacher must acknowledge that he knows the child feels different and that he understands why. "However," he tells her, "You are only different in a small way. You have [list some of her body parts that are normal] just like everyone else. And what's more, you have the same kinds of feelings that everyone else has."

It is very important for children to understand that even though their bodies are different in some way, they do not differ from other children in the nature of their feelings. Feelings become associated with traumatic medical treatments, and as a result ill children are prone to develop the idea that if their bodies are different, their feelings must be. They can develop distortions about the power of their emotions for causing further bodily harm. This idea that emotions can cause bodily harm is a hidden force, a source of emotional disturbance. It must be identified, discussed, and shown to be erroneous before it gets pushed out of awareness, buried in the unconscious mind.

Despite their sense of being different, chronically ill and handicapped children experience the same kinds of hopes, dreams, and desires that all children have. They have feelings of anger, sadness, worry, joy, and excitement just as other children do. The same kinds of things stimulate these feelings. Even though they can't *do* all the things normal children can, they wish they could. They want to have friends, join in games, and be treated as normal children despite their restrictions. They dream of becoming beautiful or admired and of gaining recognition for doing something well, the same as all children do.

EVALUATING COMPENSATORY FANTASIES

Fantasy is a useful coping mechanism, and children use it freely to cope with distressing reality. When a school-age child's fantasies become persistently discrepant with reality, adults begin to worry. They do not think it is healthy if a child who is blind in one eye truly believes he can some day have the eye exchanged for a seeing eye. They become concerned if a child whose legs are permanently paralyzed believes she will some day be able to walk. Whether any fantasy is harmful depends on whether it is aiding adjustment, facilitating personal-social development, or whether it is a sign of disturbance.

Compensatory fantasies are quite common for children who are physically disabled or who deviate from normal in some way. In their fantasies, these children perform all the feats their limitations do not allow. A girl with cerebral palsy may dream of becoming a graceful dancer; a boy with severe asthma becomes a star athlete in his fantasies; another, with stiffly jointed fingers and hands, may see himself as a successful surgeon.

The question to be asked by any concerned adult is: "How is the fantasy affecting the child's development and adjustment?" If the girl with cerebral palsy is striving to succeed in school, knows that she is liked and accepted despite her awkwardness, attends the dance recitals of her friends, and joins in games even when she is teased about her poor kicking or running, her fantasy is doing no harm and should be ignored. For such a girl, the fantasy represents a yearning for normal function, though she fully accepts herself as she is. The fantasy will either drop out or become transformed in some way as she matures. In the meantime, she obtains vicarious enjoyment by watching others perform the graceful movements that her own body cannot.

On the other hand, if the asthmatic boy, who fantasizes himself as a star athlete, is failing in school, is a social isolate who believes others don't like him, and who would rather watch TV than become involved in age-appropriate activities, he may well be in need of psychological help. His fantasy life appears to be inhibiting his intellect, restricting his interests, and causing him to withdraw and become passive toward the challenges and conflicts of growing up. He needs help, probably much more than can be given by the teacher. His apparent need for counseling should be brought to the attention of the parent, the doctor, and the school counselor.

HELPING A CHILD BUILD SELF-ESTEEM

It is common for a chronically ill child to think that he shouldn't have been born. His mental meanderings may follow any or all of the following thoughts: "I am so much trouble for everyone; my illness costs so much money; I can't become what father or mother hoped I would become; I can't do things I want to do; I must be dumb; I don't know how to make friends; nobody likes me; I am ugly (see my scars, my twisted arm, my missing leg; I'm so short; my face looks round and funny; my chest is all pushed out; I can't walk). These thoughts make the child feel that he is a burden, no good, not wanted, a disgrace, or an untouchable. Such feelings cause low esteem and contribute to a sense of inadequacy. Children with low self-esteem may believe they can't succeed in school even if they try, and they are prone to unhappy preoccupations.

Teachers and other adults need to find ways to give an ill or handicapped child a feeling that he is an important, useful, and valued person. He needs acceptance by others, but he also needs a sense of personal worth, of being valued for his unique qualities, and for what he can accomplish. Any task or way of being that is valued by others can make him feel important. For example, a cheerful, friendly disposition and a courageous spirit can be valued by others. Likewise, performing a useful task or achieving a skill through persistent effort can enhance a feeling of self-worth.

Assign Chores

Chronically ill children need chores, both at home and at school, because this is a way to be useful and helpful to others. No matter how physically restricted a child is, if he is capable of attending a regular class, he should be able to perform some kind of helpful task that will make him feel valued as a person. The list of activities should be expanded as fully as possible by teachers and parents so that children of all ages and differing capabilities can participate in doing chores. The tasks at school should not be considered privileges to be reserved for those who get work done fast. They should be distributed to all children, with some preference being given to children who have esteem problems, if this can be done without making it obvious. Other children—besides the chronically ill—who have esteem problems should be included.

Encourage Skill Development and Expertise

Developing skills or expertise of any kind makes a child feel good about himself and should be encouraged. For the child who does not excel academically or who can participate in sports in only a limited way, the teacher should think in broad ways about how the child can become expert or skilled at something. Skill in sports or dance is so heavily emphasized in some communities that other modes of activity that can help a child discover her talents are often overlooked. Chronically ill children may be unable to participate in sports and dance but may be very good at assimilating a lot of interesting information that can impress classmates and adults and stimulate conversations. Becoming adept at writing stories, drawing and art work, composing and playing music, acting, writing poetry, cooking, sewing, or doing magic tricks are among the things that should be considered when thinking of areas in which a child can develop a skill. These activities also provide emotional outlets.

Publicly Recognize Talent

Some, but not all, children need public recognition of their special abilities in order for their esteem to be boosted. The teacher can arrange for such recognition to be accorded the child. She can arrange for a display of drawings, post stories on the bulletin board, or read an exceptionally exciting child-authored story to the class. She can have a child give an oral report on an unusual topic; choose the budding actor for an important role in a play to be put on for the class, and so on. The child becomes aware of his special abilities at the same time that he is gaining recognition. Children who are shy or reserved may not wish to have their abilities touted to others. For these children, quiet signs of approval from the teacher may be all the recognition they need and want.

Children, in general, are oblivious to the fact that they have talents. They are likely to measure themselves by adult models, not realizing that, compared to other children of their own age, their special ability is not just ordinary, but outstanding. Teachers need to help children recognize their talents as a means of motivating them to develop their skills and intensify their interest in a special ability area.

Commend Interpersonal Skills

One particular kind of talent is often not recognized as such by adults: interpersonal skill. Outstanding interpersonal skills are possessed by a few children who perform them with such expertise that it is appropriate to refer to them as a talent. Interpersonal skills are not measured on tests like mental abilities and academic achievement, but they are very important for success in life. Children who have interpersonal talent perceive personal and social interactions with exceptional intuition and handle difficult situations with peers and adults in as skillful a manner as many grown-ups. When such children are suffering from low self-esteem, the teacher should let them know that their talent for dealing with people is admired by others.

Of similar importance for adjusting and getting along in life is possessing a talent for humor. When a teacher is looking for a way to make a child feel worthy, he should not overlook the significance of personal traits that are valued by others. A high capacity for humor is such a trait. Because a child's humor may be used at inappropriate times, causing the class to erupt into spasms of laughter, for example, this valuable trait is more commonly discouraged than reinforced. However, like other talents, the teacher can arrange for an amusing child to win recognition for her humor in appropriate ways.

Develop New Interests

In helping a child to expand his interests, the teacher should be alert to cues from the child. What kinds of toys does he particularly like? What kinds of books does he choose to read? What does he like to talk about? What does he draw pictures of? By watching what he does when he is free to do what he wants, the teacher can discover the child's interests.

Children grow in self-esteem, self-confidence, and socialization when they feel accepted by others. Children who are different grow best in an atmosphere where attitudes of helping, caring, and sharing are emphasized. Children become altruistic in spirit and kind and compassionate in their words and actions when adults model this kind of attitude and behavior. Children learn best when words and actions are explicit and congruent; that is, the teacher must show through actions and words that she is a caring, helping, and kind person who accepts each and every child for the person he is, if she is to expect children to model themselves after her.[2]

TEACHING ABOUT INDIVIDUAL DIFFERENCES

When children understand the physical and emotional aspects of being ill or handicapped, they are more likely to accept the child who is different. Including the subject of individual differences in the curriculum is one way of facilitating social acceptance. Acceptance is also encouraged when group projects are planned to include both handicapped and nonhandicapped students. The teacher sensitively arranges a role for the ill or handicapped child that she can perform successfully despite some specific physical, sensory, or health limitation.

Opportunities for discussing individual differences occur in nearly every curriculum area. Beginning in kindergarten, the basic concept of differentness should be developed using the children themselves, or their brothers and sisters as concrete examples. Curriculum projects to promote understanding of handicaps, both visible and invisible, should also be introduced as soon as children begin school. Topics to be developed and expanded for greater insight each year should include the impact of illness or handicap on the child and his family, his feelings about himself, and the way his life is made different by his handicap or illness.

Informal opportunities to make normal children sensitive to chronic illness and handicaps occur when children stare or ask questions about an observed difference in another child. When an ill or handicapped child is teased about his disabilities or physical differences, the teasing child should be given information rather than be scolded, and told how hurtful his remarks are for the ill or handicapped child.

USE OF LITERATURE

There are several ways in which literature can be helpful to chronically ill and handicapped children. One way involves all the children in the class and is aimed at sensitizing others to the plight of the child who is different. When healthy children read stories that foster empathy and give them information about the handicapped and chronically ill, they are more likely to be accepting of and kind to the child who is different.

Literature can also be used to help a child cope with stressful situations and unwanted facts of life. Teachers have several options in using literature for helping children cope. They can guide parents in finding helpful stories to read to their child at home; they can read stories to the class; and they can have children themselves read books and stories that are on their reading levels. When the class has been assigned to read a particular story about an ill or handicapped child, they can also be asked to write their reactions to the story. The teacher can follow this up by using the children's ideas and feelings, expressed in their themes, as the basis for a class discussion.

An annotated bibliography of books about handicaps for children and young adults, prepared by Patricia Bishopp, is available from the Meeting Street School in East Providence, Rhode Island. Another source of information is *Notes from a Different Drummer: A Guide to Juvenile Fiction Portraying the Handicapped* (Barbara Baskin and Karen Harris, R. R. Bowker, NY, 1977). This book has an annotated bibliography but also discusses things to consider in using this type of literature. Joan Fassler's book, *Helping Children Cope: Mastering Stress through Books* (The Free Press, NY, 1978) discusses the content of some of the best books that are useful to children faced with a variety of stressful situations. Fassler also proposes questions to stimulate a discussion for children who have heard the stories. She discusses books that help build personal courage, stories about illness and pain, stories having to do with loneliness and self-esteem problems, books helpful to the hospitalized child, and books that have to do with achieving a sense of independence and autonomy. Fassler's book is oriented toward the younger age group, while the other annotated bibliographies are oriented toward the older age group.

COPING WITH THE CURIOSITY OF OTHER CHILDREN

Children are curious; but curiosity about the handicapped or ill child is something of a taboo in our society. In large measure, a child does not feel that it is appropriate to express curiosity in this area. If he does express it, his curiosity is not likely to be satisfied. Adults either do not know the answers to the child's questions or say they do not, because they feel anxious or constrained.

Children learn very early in life, at a subconscious level, from the subtle cues of their elders not to show an interest in or curiosity about the different child. In their effort to understand, they may imitate what they see: the spastic gait, the slurred or stuttering speech, the gasping breath, the convulsion, and the like. They may put blindfolds over their eyes or cotton in their ears in an effort to experience the world of the blind or deaf. When they are discovered by an adult who thinks they are mocking the different child, they are embarrassed and laugh it off. The myth is that children are cruel because it is always assumed that normal children are making fun of the child who looks, walks, or talks in an unusual way.

Studies have shown that children as young as age two can behave altruistically.[3] It would seem that children's natural tendencies are to be interested in and helpful to others. They are not, by nature, cruel and do not need to be unkind. It is true that if curiosity is permitted, the ill child will be confronted with stares and questions by well children. The incidence of unkind actions will be minimal, I believe, if well or normal children's curiosities are satisfied.

The ill child needs to be able to respond to the stares and questions of other children with equanimity. He can learn to do this if he has a simple statement he can make that explains his condition, when others act curious. If a child's doctor has not taught him such a statement, the teacher or parent should do so. The statement should be in specific and honest words that are appropriate to the child's level of understanding.[4]

The following statements are quoted from the pamphlet, *The Chronically Ill Child and Family in the Community*. They can serve as a model in framing statements for less common conditions. Teachers and parents who feel uneasy about framing a statement for an illness not illustrated should consult the child's doctor.

- *For diabetes:* "I have diabetes—that means my body doesn't use sugar the same ways yours does. That's why I take shots and watch what I eat."

- *For chemotherapy with cancer:* "I was really sick when I was in the hospital. The medicine they gave me for my cancer made my hair fall out. It'll grow back. I'll sure be glad when it does."

- *For cystic fibrosis:* "I get this stuff in my lungs that makes me cough a lot—when I do cough it up, I can breathe better. I have stomach problems but I take pills which help me digest my food."

- *For cerebral palsy:* "My muscles don't get the right messages to make them move the way I want them to. These metal things are braces. I wear them to help my legs. Some kids wear braces on their teeth."

- *For asthma:* "I have asthma and that means my lungs give me trouble stometimes. If I get excited or if the air is dirty and full of dust, I have trouble breathing and I wheeze like this. As long as I take my medicine, I'm usually okay."

- *For hemophilia:* "I have to be careful because I have hemophilia. You know how when you get a cut, it bleeds a little and then dries up? Well, my blood has a hard time drying up and I bleed a lot. It's not good to lose a lot of blood, so I have to be careful."

- *For a heart defect:* "There are a lot of parts of your heart that work to make it run, sort of like a car engine. Some of the parts of mine don't work as well as others."

- *For mental retardation:* "School is really hard for me even when I try hard. I have brain damage and that means it's hard for me to do things as fast as you, even when I try hard."

- *For seizures:* "Your brain tells your arms and legs how to work. Sometimes my brain gets the message wrong and my arms and legs and whole body shake. When that happens, just leave me alone. I'll be okay in a minute. It's not catching. Most of the time, the medicine I take helps prevent the shaking."

- *For spina bifida:* "I was born with a part of my back still open and the doctors had to do an operation to close it. Because of that I have trouble walking and have to use special crutches. I like to do the same things you do, but I can't run."

- A child can say: "Everybody's different—some of us have differences that show on the outside, and others have differences which are on the inside."
- The child may need to reassure other children that the condition is not catching.*

HELPING WITH SOCIALIZATION

Many chronically ill children miss out on important socialization experiences. Their life experiences have been different from those of well children and they may not "speak the same language." They may not be able to join in the running, rough-and-tumble play of their peers. They may be shy and uncertain of how to make friends. Because of their sense of isolation, they may remain aloof, out of fear of being rejected. They may not have game-playing or physical skills comparable to their peers. They may have continuing needs to play at a less mature level than their peers. Their parents may not be doing all that is possible to encourage social experience.

Teachers usually try to help the child who is socially isolated by suggesting to other children that they invite him to join their play. They will also urge the loner himself to make his wants known when he wishes to be included by others. However, sometimes the usual and ordinary efforts to get a child socially involved fail. It may be that he is not ready for social participation at his age level. Helping him join the play of younger children may be an answer, if it is the nature of his behavior and type of play he prefers that is the barrier between him and his age-mates.

However, some children need to recapitulate the sequences of normal social growth in order to feel able to make friends and to participate in group activities. Parents may need to be reminded and encouraged to take the child through these steps also.

When a child needs to be taken through the sequences of social growth, the teacher must first become a trusted, nurturing person. Then, careful arrangement of one-to-one social contacts with another child should take place with an adult present. (Parents can be advised to invite a child to come for a visit along with her parent.) The child chosen to be the first friend may be another isolate, or she may be a

---

*Quoted from *The Chronically Ill Child and Family in the Community*, published by the Association for the Care of Children's Health, 1982. Used by permission.

particularly empathetic child who is easily drawn toward a needy person. The teacher should look for spontaneous cues of attraction between the poorly socialized ill child and a classmate. With a sense of having one friend, feelings of being alone and rejected can begin to diminish. If the child is lacking in the social skills of give-and-take, sharing, winning and losing, and playing according to the rules, these will need to be developed in the one-to-one relationship. As the child feels more confident in relating to others, she will begin to participate more fully and enthusiastically in small group activities within the classroom.

From formally constituted group activities within the classroom, under supervision, the child may be ready to join small informal play groups that form on the playground. At this point, she may be invited to a classmate's party and gradually start moving in and out of friendships with several children. It will take a long time, perhaps several years, for some children to attain the social level of their age-mates. They may continue to harbor a sensitivity to rejection for a very long time.

ALTERNATIVES TO COMPETITION

The chronically ill child is at a disadvantage regarding competition. Chronic illness often restricts the kind or vigorousness of physical activity that a child may engage in. Competition, which can cause a child to overstress himself physically, should be eliminated as an aspect of physical activity. The teacher should consider alternatives to competition. This principle applies to academic competition as well as to competition in sports. (Academic competition is discussed in Chapter 6.)

Individual Sports

Individual kinds of physical activity, such as swimming, skiing, hiking, and bicycling, are alternatives to competitive sports. These are also good for the children who have not yet reached the social developmental stage of being able to play games according to rules. For some children, these may be the only kinds of physical activity allowed.

Cooperative Games

Cooperative games are an alternative to competitive sports. In a cooperative game, children are provided with challenges while playing with, rather than against, each other. This kind of game is a way to promote acceptance and sharing, as well as cooperation. Feelings of failure are eliminated, and no one has to worry about measuring up. A child's confidence in himself can be reinforced at the same time that he is having fun and feeling accepted. In this way, self-esteem is enhanced.

Terry Orlick's book, *The Cooperative Sports and Games Book*, describes many cooperative games for all ages. Both active games, requiring a lot of space, and quiet indoor games are included. Some of the games require gymnasium equipment; others use simpler props.

Of particular interest in Orlick's book is the section on inventing new games. Orlick has worked with groups of children, asking them to create new games or to improve on old ones to make them more fun. The only requirements he stipulated were that the children must stick to the principles of cooperative games: Everyone must participate; children should be helpful to one another; everyone is to have fun; no one is to feel like a loser. The children enjoyed the process of creation. They worked in small groups. This, in itself, promoted social interaction, decision making, and accommodating one's ideas to the wishes of the group.

Orlick also reminds the reader that competitive sports—where only the few best can play, where players are eliminated, and where there is a lot of "putting down" for goofs and errors—are adult concepts. Self-organized games by kids usually put more emphasis on having fun than on winning.*

NOTES

1. Elizabeth McAnarney and others, "Psychological Problems of Children with Chronic Juvenile Arthritis," *Pediatrics* 53:525, 1974, p. 526.

2. Paul Mussen and Nancy Eisenberg-Berg, *The Roots of Caring, Sharing, and Helping* (San Francisco: W. H. Freeman, 1977) pp. 74–100.

3. Maya Pines, "Good Samaritans at Age Two?", *Psychology Today*, June 1979, pp. 66–77.

4. *The Chronically Ill Child and Family in the Community* (Pamphlet) (Washington, DC: Association for the Care of Children's Health, 1982) pp. 17–18.

---

*Adapted from *The Cooperative Sports and Games Book* by Terry Orlick, published by Pantheon Books, © 1978 by Terry Orlick. Used by permission.

5

How to Help Children Adjust When Chronic Illness Affects Social and Emotional Development

> Ronald had gotten the idea that he had special powers. "Yeh, that's gotta be it," he told himself, "because anyone with any brains can see that all I need to do is wish for something and it appears. And do you know what? Every time I have to be in the hospital my folks stop fighting! They are so nice it is sort of sickening. So how come my special powers don't work in school? How come I have to do all that work?"

Children with chronic illness are at a much higher risk for the development of social and emotional problems than are other children. Indeed, the incidence of problems in the chronically ill group is two to three times greater than in the general population.[1] This chapter discusses how and why a chronically ill child develops emotional and behavioral problems, and shows what steps a teacher can take to deal with them.

OVERPROTECTIVENESS

Children need protection, and they need it even more when they are sick. It is often difficult for parents to realize or accept that they are being overprotective. Being overly protective means prohibiting a child from having experiences that facilitate healthy social and emotional development. The experiences that a parent restricts may be perceived as potentially harmful in either a physical or emotional sense. For example, a child with hemophilia may not be allowed any physical activity, out of fear of precipitating a bleeding episode. The psychological and social consequences of this may be more harmful than the bleeding episode. In any event, bleeding episodes often occur spontaneously, without the child being bumped. Another child may be kept from joining the scouts, some social group, or a special-interest club because a parent feels he will be teased, rejected, or otherwise suffer embarrassment. In this case, the parent is trying to protect the child from emotional hurts.

The child who is overprotected develops a heightened sense of vulnerability. Fears become intensified, and she may withdraw at the slightest hint of a difficult situation. She is likely to be either excessively shy or boldly demanding. She will most certainly lack confidence, as she has never had to handle situations on her own. Her mother or father will rush to the school with complaints or demands whenever a problem occurs.

Parents who are overprotective believe they are acting in their child's best interests. As they have had to relinquish a degree of their parental authority to doctors and nurses, they have perhaps become overly zealous about carrying out their protective functions because they have felt displaced to some extent by medical personnel. Commonly, though, they are overly protective because of their intense anxiety. They fear that something worse might happen to their child, or they can't bear to see their child hurt or rejected by other children.

In guiding parents to change their pathogenic attitude and the unhealthy practices associated with it, it is important to avoid telling them they are overprotective. Instead, you should explain how their parenting is interfering with their child's growth. Parents want to do what's right for their child. If they are unduly restrictive, they must be helped to see how this is affecting the child's development. It is likely that both the doctor and the teacher will be concerned. It would be wise for them to consult with one another before discussing this matter with the parents. If the father can see the harm of overprotecting, and the mother can't, efforts can be made to get the father to influence the mother. The child's efforts to stand on his own must also be reinforced, and he must continually be reassured that his illness is not likely to become worse. This latter reassurance requires the participation of the doctor.

OVERINDULGENCE AND THE IMPORTANCE OF DISCIPLINE

When a child's every whim is catered to; when he is waited on hand and foot although he is capable of doing things for himself; when little is required of him in the way of family duty; and when he is allowed to do whatever he pleases, even if his behavior encroaches on the rights of others, he will become an extremely overindulged child. His personality will fail to mature, and he will remain a demanding, dictatorial, controlling adult. He will find it difficult to make friends, as few people will tolerate his self-centered demands. He will rebel against rules in the classroom, as he has never been governed by rules at home. He will have little patience for waiting, or little tolerance for frustration.

Parents often exempt the ill child from the expectations, limitations, and rules that they have for their normal children. This kind of indulging arises out of their sympathy for the ill child and from their own anguish that they are powerless to make him well and healthy. Ill children who are indulged, pampered, catered to, and allowed to get away with anything are undisciplined. They are resented by siblings and are usually poorly adjusted.

A child who is not disciplined or held accountable for living up to the behavioral standards set for her brothers and sisters knows she is perceived by others as being different. Even though this mark of being different is not in her best interests, she may bask in it and take advantage of her "privileged" position. It is not good for a chronically ill child to have her sense of differentness confirmed by being exempted from discipline.

The most effective discipline is based on helping a child behave according to the accepted standards for a child his age. Whether he is ill or well, parents have to teach their child to obey, require him to adhere to rules, and expect increasing levels of independence and responsibility from him as he matures. They must prevent him from wrongdoing by setting firm limits.

Discipline means behavioral self-control. Parents do not have to give much conscious attention to disciplinary measures as such when they help their child to act correctly. Instead, this can be accomplished by setting firm limits on aggressive impulses and on tendencies of the child to be intrusive or obtrusive; by making sure that chores are assigned and carried out; and by teaching the principle of mutual respect as the basis for interpersonal relating. The term *mutual respect* means that each family member is respected in his right to pursue his own satisfactions and achieve mastery at his own age level, until that pursuit infringes on the rights of other family members to do the same. This form of positive behavioral training, which almost eliminates the need to think in terms of punishment, is desirable for all children, but particularly so for chronically ill children. Teachers and parents must adhere to these principles of discipline with the chronically ill child.

Parents who cannot conceive of a wheelchair-bound child doing chores should be helped to imagine all the useful things their child can do with the hands, eyes, and mouth. Only a severely crippled child who has no functional use of any appendages should be exempted from chores.

OVERINVOLVEMENT: A SYMBIOTIC RELATIONSHIP

A mother (and occasionally a father) may become intensely emotionally involved with a chronically ill child. The overattachment is a kind of fusion in which the mother experiences her child's pain and emotions as if they were her own. The child fails to learn to separate himself from his mother. He may seem almost able to read her mind in that he senses her anxiety and fear, guesses her thoughts, and is hyperalert to all cues and nonverbal messages from her. The mother has the same kinds of responses. Mother and child become mutually interdependent in terms of taking care of each other's emotions. There is a powerful force of emotional transmission between them. They do not feel comfortable when apart from each other. The intensity of their emotional bonding restricts their relationships with others. The father tends to feel left out and becomes distant. The child fails to make friends and does not become involved with peers. This kind of parental reaction has serious consequences for a child's social and emotional development. Psychotherapy for the family will most likely be necessary.

PSYCHOSOMATIC EXACERBATION OF CHRONIC ILLNESS

When illness occurs in the body, the mind responds by giving the person a sense of not feeling well. Feelings of weakness, malaise, pain, and so on, are all aspects of the general mental event of not feeling well. What happens to the body affects the feelings and mood.

A reverse process can also take place. Emotions, such as fear, anger, and sadness, can set in motion physical changes in heart rate, breathing, glandular secretions, and vascularity. When the emotional reaction is of sufficient intensity or duration, physical symptoms such as pain, vomiting, diarrhea, and others, result. In this case, what starts as a mental event—the experiencing of strong emotions—leads to physical symptoms suggestive of illness.

Mind and body have a powerful influence on each other. The relationship between illness and emotions has been recognized for a long time. In fact, before the recent explosion of medical and scientific knowledge revealed the true cause and mechanisms of illnesses, a number of illnesses were thought to be caused by emotional factors. Asthma, juvenile rheumatoid arthritis, and juvenile diabetes mellitus are among such illnesses. Many people still believe that asthma can be caused by emotional factors, although it is quite clear that a person must have an asthmatic lung in order to respond to emotional events with an asthmatic attack. Emotions can trigger an attack of asthma, and emotions can trigger attacks or episodes of other illnesses, such as epilepsy or diabetes; but the illness is not *caused* by emotional factors.

Psychosomatic is the word used to refer to the mind-body relationship. Perhaps the most commonly understood meaning of psychosomatic is that physical symptoms of illness are considered to have originated from emotional conflicts. For example, a person who is not dealing with an emotional conflict satisfactorily may develop a headache, stomachache, or ulcer. *Psychosomatic* also defines the mind-body interactions in organic diseases. When emotional factors bring on an attack of a preexisting physical illness or make the medical condition of the illness worse, the illness has developed into a psychosomatic condition. In this instance, a medical illness *becomes* psychosomatic because psychological factors are setting in motion physiological processes that exacerbate the medical problem.

Any illness has the potential to become psychosomatic. When it does, the medical condition will be hard to manage, the doctor will be worried and feel frustrated, and parental anxiety will increase. The doctor usually presumes that emotional factors are an important concern when a child is not responding as expected to medical treatment. This is not always an accurate presumption, as certain illnesses are known to be capricious. Juvenile diabetes mellitus, juvenile rheumatoid arthritis, and hemophilia all have periods of exacerbation and calm, often without explanation or known causes.

Professionals dealing with chronically ill children and their families must be alert to the environmental factors that pose a threat to the ill child. Children react to family tension. They also react emotionally to situations in school and to those involving their peers.

Many factors within the home and—as the child and family interact—in the outside world contribute to an illness becoming psychosomatic. For this reason, diagnostic and therapeutic approaches should include the family and take into consideration the environment, including the school, not just the individual child.

Tension in the Home

Family tension can arise from communication breakdowns and relationship difficulties among family members (including extended family): from the manner in which conflict is dealt with or avoided and from other factors such as economic difficulties, crowded conditions, or natural disasters. A high level of family tension causes a home climate that can produce a range of adjustment difficulties and psychosomatic illness. The following example illustrates this.

There was a great deal of tension in Diane's family.

> Diane is an eight-year-old diabetic. Her brother is five years old. Diane was hospitalized four times for ketoacidosis during the past six months and is a worry to her doctor, who now considers her diabetes to have developed into a psychosomatic problem.
>
> A family interview reveals that Diane interrupts her parents' conversations frequently. She answers questions addressed to her brother, and she interferes with his play. She bosses him, telling him what he can and cannot do. Her parents have not set limits on her intrusiveness. In addition, they allow her to make most of the decisions in the family.
>
> Her parents have been informed by the school that Diane does her work only sporadically, seemingly only when she feels like it. They express a feeling of impotence in regard to getting Diane to do what her teacher expects.
>
> Her father and mother disagree about how to handle Diane, but they pretend to be in accord. Her mother does not want to set limits because she fears the diabetes will get worse; her father accepts her mother's permissive view and collaborates by doing nothing. However, he feels resentful about Diane's domination of the family and distances himself by staying at work for long hours. Family tension is at such a high level that both parents wonder if divorce would be a solution. It seems apparent that when the family tension reaches a peak, Diane develops ketoacidosis and is hospitalized. The parents pull together to get her condition stabilized, and this deescalates the anxiety level in the family; but nothing changes.
>
> The cycle of family tension, Diane's diabetes going out of control in reaction to it, parents pulling together, deescalation of anxiety for a short time, and then gradual build-up of family tension again repeats itself over and over.

Salvador Minuchin and others have identified a pattern of family organization that is characteristic of families where a child's illness becomes psychosomatic.[2] In these families, members are overprotective of each other and they lack flexibility in dealing with problems. They avoid conflict because any potential conflict creates too much anxiety. The sick child, by becoming sicker when the family tension increases (because they cannot bring their differences out into the open), plays an important role in helping the family avoid conflict. Minuchin believes that family psychotherapy is the treatment that has the most chance of success with a child whose illness has become psychosomatic.

Tension in the School

When a teacher has too high or too rigid a set of expectations, fails to recognize a learning disability, or is highly critical or deprecating of children, it is possible that school-based factors can contribute to a child's psychosomatic problem. This was the case with Adam.

> Adam was a twelve-year-old seventh grader who had asthma. He had learned and adjusted satisfactorily until he reached junior high school. Now the demands of large amounts of homework, combined with critical remarks from teachers, made him fearful of failing. His asthma, previously under control, suddenly became worse. His morning wheezing was severe enough that he was allowed to stay home. Missed schoolwork piled up, increasing his sense of being overwhelmed. Overuse of a broncho-dilator (to reduce the wheezing) made him hyperactive and unable to concentrate, further compounding his difficulties and increasing his fear of failing.
>
> Attention to the school problem was necessary to reverse the process. A Child Study Evaluation showed him to have adequate skills and abilities to achieve success. No serious family problems were revealed; mild social anxiety related to peer relationships was evident. The school counselor became active as a liaison between Adam and his teachers, talked with the doctor about medication and use of the broncho-dilator, and began seeing Adam for weekly counseling sessions. His parents arranged for a tutor to give him help and support until missed work was made up.

EMOTIONAL PROBLEMS AFFECTING OVERALL ADJUSTMENT

Psychosomatic exacerbation of illness is but one way that a chronically ill child expresses strong emotions such as fear and anger. The difficulties created for a child by her illness and those created by the way peers and other adults treat her or react to her also cause emotional trouble. Emotional problems in sick children may be expressed in the same manner as in healthy children; that is, emotional conflicts of both chronically ill and healthy children are expressed by failing in school, by unwarranted aggression toward others, by extreme passivity and withdrawal, by acting like a child several years younger, and by acting unusually provocative or "crazy," and so on. This kind of emotional problem resides within the child but is created by forces outside of himself over which he has no control. In treating this kind of emotional problem, the environmental factors must be given important consideration. If the environmental factors stem primarily from the school situation, intervention by the school counselor may be the way to start. If the family situation is a major source of conflict for the child, family-focused counseling would be most appropriate. If the child is dealing with conflicts primarily related to the illness itself, individual help or group counseling with other children having the same or another chronic illness may be the therapeutic approach that would be most beneficial.

Home and School Factors

The following story about Sharon illustrates how factors in both the home and school interlocked to produce symptoms that made Sharon appear to be much more emotionally disturbed than she actually was.

> Sharon was a twelve-year-old who had mild cerebral palsy and grand mal epilepsy. However, the correct diagnoses were not made until she was six years old, when her seizures started. Prior to this, the family had been told during her infancy that Sharon had a rare syndrome that would cause her to be moderately to severely retarded. They had lowered their expectations dramatically and treated her as if she were retarded.
>
> With the change in diagnosis, her parents began to believe that Sharon might have normal intelligence, as the new doctor suggested this was possible. Sharon began to act much smarter as soon as the parents started expecting more. She started school and made slow but normal progress in learning how to read, spell, write, and calculate. She began having trouble in fourth grade because of difficulties with language (not diagnosed until much later).
>
> In fifth grade, an IQ test classified her as of borderline retarded intelligence. She remained in a regular class, but now everyone (including her parents) treated her as though she were

retarded. It was puzzling, though, that her performance in some areas was quite average. Clearly, teachers and parents thought, she wasn't retarded but was not trying hard enough (in the subjects with which she was having trouble).

Actually, Sharon had a learning disability involving the comprehension and expression of complex language structures. She misunderstood directions and even misunderstood interpersonal communication exchanges when there was strong emotion attached. Her parents became very protective of her when she had problems at school with teachers and with learning, believing that the teachers were not kind or helpful. They began to vacillate in the way they treated Sharon. Sometimes they treated her as if she were retarded, sometimes as if she were 100 percent normal. She was neither.

Sharon had difficulties with her self-image and in acting like a normal girl of twelve. She had serious relationship difficulties. She withdrew from engaging in activities outside of the home, was extremely dependent on her mother, and had tantrums when asked to do family chores. Sharon's emotional eruptions, her rebellious attitude, and the degree of her social withdrawal all suggested severe emotional disturbance. However, by obtaining a psychological evaluation that clarified the nature of the problem, focusing on changing the parental and family reactions and changing the way her learning and communication difficulties were dealt with at school, Sharon soon "lost" many of the symptoms that were an expression of her emotional dilemmas and of everyone else's confusion about what to expect of her and how to treat her.

Emotional Effects of Cerebral Palsy

A child with cerebral palsy is quite vulnerable to developing social and emotional difficulties even if parental vacillation, protectiveness, and misdiagnosis are not aspects of the situation, as with Sharon. Sharon had only a twisted hand, a mildly uneven gait, and an occasional slurring of speech as observable features of her cerebral palsy. However, many children with cerebral palsy have a more pronounced appearance. The child with cerebral palsy may drool, move his mouth awkwardly in an effort to talk, or have slurred or inarticulate speech. He may have a twisted hand or wear a leg brace. He may lurch, jerk, or wave his arms at random. The immediate image created in the minds of other children is that of a drunk or a retarded person. A seven-year-old whose gait and hand movements were reminiscent of feminine gestures and walking was even called *gay*. (The children did not know he had cerebral palsy.)

Children who experience rejection and ridicule from others may become shy and withdrawn or strike out with hostility. These children frequently don't report experiences of being made fun of. Their embarrassment and sense of inferiority—but most of all their hope of eventual acceptance—prompt them to keep such experiences to themselves. The more sensitive and less bold cerebral palsy children may become frightened of being alone with other children. They have learned that the presence of an adult will assure that they will not be hurt and that ridicule will be minimized. By requiring the presence of an adult, they are perceived by others as being dependent and immature, and this puts even greater distance between themselves and their peers. It also causes some adults to react negatively to them.

Social and behavioral difficulties can arise for a child with cerebral palsy with a severe speech problem because he cannot make himself understood. He may also misunderstand the meaning of what others say to him, as receptive difficulty, particularly of complex language, is common.

Emotional Effects of Epilepsy

Epilepsy is another disorder that makes a child particularly vulnerable to developing social and emotional problems.[3] Epilepsy carries with it a social onus that causes others to avoid contact and exclude the child from social groups. The uncontrolled twitching and contorted movements of generalized seizures are frightening to both children and adults.

Seizures are now being classified into two major groups: generalized and nongeneralized. Generalized seizures begin by involving both hemispheres of the brain. They include *grand mal* and *petit mal* seizures. Nongeneralized seizures begin by involving one of the two hemispheres. The nongeneralized seizures are further divided into two categories called *simple partial,* which does not impair consciousness, and *complex partial,* which may impair thinking and consciousness. These latter seizures include those called *temporal lobe* and *psychomotor.*

Unusual behaviors before and after a seizure (ictus), reflecting the pre-ictal and post-ictal states, are also troubling to others. During these states, a child may have hallucinations, act confused, or say or do odd things. The child may have difficulty understanding spoken language and may have difficulty speaking, have memory lapses, and exhibit changes in emotionality.[4] Epilepsy occurs in a significant proportion of children with cerebral palsy. Thus, children with both cerebral palsy and epilepsy are doubly vulnerable to developing a psychological disorder.

How the Teacher Can Help

A child who is in a post-ictal state (he could have sustained a seizure at home the night before or during sleep) will be confused. He will need help in focusing his attention. He may need a lot of reorienting and structure. With such a child, the teacher should stand nearby and help him find the correct page, make a brief statement about what the lesson is about, and be ready to give him additional directions and explanations once the class has started on its work. If a seizure occurs during the school day, the child may need time away from the class to lie down and sleep. He should be asked if he wants to go to the nurse's office to lie down.

A teacher must be aware that epileptic seizures have many variations. Epilepsy is not always diagnosed until a child has had it for some time. It is rare for a child to have hallucinations unless there is something wrong with his brain, and yet a child with hallucinations is sometimes sent to a mental health clinic rather than to a medical doctor. Seizures are sometimes not caused by epilepsy but are the early symptoms of a more serious occurrence in the brain such as a brain tumor, lead poisoning, stroke, or an acute illness such as meningitis.

BEHAVIOR DISORDERS

Children who act up, act out, who do not mind, or do not behave in accord with the established rules, are referred to as having a behavior or conduct disorder. These children are very distressing to parents and teachers. Appropriate management of such children depends on correct diagnosis regarding the basis of the behavior disorder. Behavioral difficulties may be either psychologically based or may be the expression of an organic disorder.

Psychological Origin

A behavior disorder may be the expression of an emotional problem; that is, a child may ignore rules because of rebellious feelings; he may disrupt the class to focus attention on himself; or he may clown and act foolish to relieve himself of burdensome expectations that he cannot meet. A psychologically based behavior disorder may also be the result of a learned way to react to specific stimuli. For example, the child who has learned that having a tantrum or acting badly gets him what he wants, may continue to act badly in all situations where he is denied anything. When a chronically ill child has a behavior disorder correctly diagnosed as an expression of an emotional problem, or as a learned way to respond to specific situations or interactions, psychological intervention in one form or another is indicated.

Even when counseling for a child or his family seems the most logical way to help him become better behaved, it is often not easy to get parents to proceed with it. The school continues to have the problem of what to do with a child who acts out. Exclusion from school is no longer a solution. What can the teacher do?

First, it is important to be sure that the behavior problem is indeed psychological in origin rather than an aspect of an organic disorder. The teacher should refer the child for a complete evaluation by the school's special services staff (see Chapter 12). The evaluation will not only establish the basis of the problem (if organicity is suspected, the child will be referred for further medical and psychiatric evaluation), but it should also offer some clues about how to deal with the child. A teacher should not expect to know how to deal with a serious behavior disorder without advice and support from other professionals. Her source of help can be the school counselor or psychologist, a special education teacher who has a class of behavior-disordered children, or a mental health professional from outside the school. If the special services staff believes the child's problems are severe enough, a special class may be recommended.

With psychologically based behavior problems, disciplinary actions—in cooperation with the principal, when necessary—are appropriate. If problems persist despite repeated use of disciplinary procedures, the parents must be informed. The way the problem is reported to parents is important. An accurate statement of what the child did or said—and perhaps how many times it happened and what was tried to correct the problem—should be given without making any interpretations, accusations, judgments, or threats. The teacher must stick to facts. He should ask parents for suggestions about how to deal with the child's behavior, and how the parents see themselves working with the school to find a solution. Some parents will need to be specifically told that they must impress on their child that she must behave in school. This may need to be done by the principal, whose authority carries more weight.

Organic Origin

Behavior disorders that are the result of brain dysfunction, temporal lobe epilepsy, or any of a number of other medical disorders or medical treatments are called *organic behavior disorders.* They require a different understanding. Different approaches to management are required. The differentiation between psychologically based and organically based behavior disorders requires the collaboration of a psychologist and a physician. A child psychiatrist who has maintained an interest in and contact with general medicine may be an appropriate professional to consult. Pediatricians and neurologists who incorporate results of a Child Study Evaluation done by a school, clinic, or private psychologist into their diagnostic data base can also correctly distinguish between the two kinds of behavior disorders.

Medications that are taken to manage or treat a medical condition can cause a variety of reactions. Among these are hyperactivity, tremors, lethargy, and personality change with accompanying difficult behavior. When hyperactivity or unusual behaviors are believed to be the result of medications, appropriate evaluation by the physician is necessary. Teachers may be asked to record the time when the behavior occurs to establish whether or not it is related to medication intake.

Nature of Organic Behavior Disorders

When a child's brain has been involved in illness or he has suffered some kind of insult to the brain at birth or later, he is likely to have some degree of behavior disorder.

The term *organic behavior disorder* means that behaviors labeled *inappropriate, unusual, undesirable,* or *unpredictable* are presumed not to be under the control of the child. The behaviors "happen" for seemingly inexplicable reasons. Until proven otherwise, a behavior disorder should be assumed to be organic in nature when there has been some antecedent event that could have involved the brain.

Behavior difficulties following insults to the brain include temper tantrums, impulsiveness, outbursts of aggression, lack of judgment, impaired perception of social cues, and poor ability to adapt to new situations. When cognitive impairment has also occurred as a result of the brain insult, behavioral difficulties may be of greater magnitude.

Effect of Viral Illness

Severe viral illness may have affected brain function without anyone being aware of it. Very high fevers of unknown origin are an example. Ben had been hospitalized for a severe illness, although the illness had not been given a name.

Ben was seen at age ten, having suffered a severe viral illness with very high fevers at age five. He attained a normal verbal IQ on an intelligence scale and could read, write, spell, and calculate at grade level. However, he could not answer questions in a logical, direct manner, and could not construct a written theme that made sense. He could not make up stories with a logical or sensible sequence of ideas. He showed a lack of judgment in his everyday behavior and did not understand social cues. Despite his normal IQ, he was a misfit socially and could not master higher-level learning. He showed signs of brain dysfunction on special tests. Ben's problems proved to be so severe that he first went to a special class within the regular school and later to a special school. Despite his normal verbal IQ, he functioned cognitively as a mildly retarded boy.

Additional Medical Causes

Unusual and difficult behavior may reflect a previously undiagnosed medical problem such as a brain tumor, lead poisoning, or temporal lobe epilepsy. Rarer disorders such as Gilles de la Tourette's disease and Wilson's disease are also marked by unusual behaviors.

Ralph's unusual behavior reflected an undiagnosed medical problem that required immediate surgical intervention.

> Ralph had been a normal boy until second grade. Now he began to demonstrate a number of peculiar behaviors: feeling the walls, getting lost, going to his locker without asking, hiding under tables, and so on. He had had two seizures during the summer and was put on medication for epilepsy. As his unusual behavior continued, the school asked for a psychological evaluation. The organic findings on a number of tests and the inexplicable nature of his behavior pointed to a need for medical evaluation. He was subsequently diagnosed as having a brain tumor.

In temporal lobe epilepsy, the pre-seizure (pre-ictal) and post-seizure (post-ictal) states may last for hours or days. Pre-ictally, the child may experience strange sensations and a sense of fear prompting him to run, as well as hallucinations that can be vivid and unpleasant. The seizure itself may vary greatly from child to child but tends to take a similar form for a particular child. Complex, coordinated but *purposeless,* motor movements occur (for example, lip smacking or walking in a circle, with a blank stare or stereotyped verbalizations). Any repeated, stereotyped, and meaningless behavior may reflect a temporal lobe seizure. Although the seizure itself is of short duration (probably no longer than one minute), the post-ictal state can be quite long. A state of confusion, headache, or a feeling of exhaustion enough to want to sleep, occur post-ictally. Combativeness and violent behavior may occur during this post-ictal confusional period, especially if a well-meaning observer attempts to help or restrain the person.[5]

The Need for Medical Evaluation

It is unwise to assume that a child who develops tics, seems to be hallucinating, or otherwise acts peculiarly has a psychiatric problem. These children should always be referred to a medical doctor for evaluation. Children with intractable, very difficult behavior also need to be thoroughly evaluated medically.

Multidisciplinary clinics in hospital settings are appropriate places to refer children who have unusual behavior. These clinics are likely to be in the pediatrics department of a general hospital. At such a clinic, a child will receive a thorough medical evaluation and an assessment of learning and emotional factors.

Brain Damage from Head Injury

Children who have suffered brain damage as a result of head injury usually have a difficult time adjusting. Their problems are quite different from those of children with cerebral palsy. Although both have suffered brain damage that has probably affected their physical capabilities, their ability to communicate satisfactorily and ability to learn, the time of the occurrence of brain damage is a distinguishing factor. Cerebral palsy brain injury occurs prenatally, at birth, or during the neonatal period. Accidental head injury resulting in brain damage that occurs during the growing-up years will affect personality and intellect that are already formed. The later it occurs, the greater will be its impact. The older child and adolescent will suffer personality change that may be too dismaying to grasp, either by himself or by others.[6] The great change in his behavior will be bewildering. Brain damage may cause loss of some of his old learning, but not all. This results in a discontinuity of his experience, which is continually upsetting to him. It causes him to feel unstable; he has difficulty predicting whether or not he can master a learning task or cope with a social situation.

The older child or adolescent who suffers brain damage may have had high aspirations and commensurate abilities to reach them prior to the accident. Her lofty goals may be retained while the capacity to attain them has been lost. Parents may think that their child's or adolescent's change in behavior is only a problem of discipline and fail to appreciate the magnitude of the emotional devastation that is experienced when functions are lost or partially disrupted. Medical personnel may become angry and frustrated when an older child or adolescent will not cooperate with their rehabilitative efforts. The depression resulting from loss of capacities can be expressed by marked withdrawal or aggressive acting out in response to efforts to help her recover her capacities to the fullest extent possible.

The post-brain damage behavior of the older child or adolescent suffering head injury comprises lack of judgment, bewilderment, inability to cope with frustration, and depression. These personality factors are not aspects of the cerebral palsy child's emotional problems, although the cerebral palsy child has the more generalized difficulties cited earlier.

Management of Organic Behavior Disorders

If behavior and learning difficulties resulting from brain damage are not correctly recognized as organic in origin, the teacher and parents can become frustrated by use of the wrong techniques, and the child's behavioral difficulties may become worse. Management, rather than discipline, is the guiding principle to be applied.

Management approaches for the child who has an organic behavior disorder center around behavior modification strategies and environmental manipulation, which reflect the principles of social learning theory. Inability to sort out stimuli can be confusing to a brain-damaged child and also make concentrating on a task difficult. A great deal of structure, aids for focusing of attention, and provision for limitation of distracting elements will be important considerations. The child may need to use a carrel in order to be able to concentrate on his work in school. The teacher should maintain a very clear and consistent structure in the classroom. She should also give the child a written list of essential rules (with perhaps an accompanying graphic cue for each one). A chart for reinforcing adherence to rules can also be made, with stars, checks, or some other symbol put on the chart when the child follows a rule that he habitually tends to forget.

Teachers (and also parents) must remain alert to behavioral cues in communicating with children with brain dysfunction. A child's behavior will indicate whether or not he is responding to a message as intended. A child with brain dysfunction may not attend to or remember verbal cues. Also, such a child may repeat the verbal message but may not be able to translate it correctly in behavioral terms. This kind of child may have to be shown what to do so that he can respond through imitation.

Environmental Manipulation

    Environmental manipulation means that certain aspects of the home or learning situation are changed to accommodate the difficulties a child has in sorting out stimuli, remembering rules, or controlling behavior. The special class is a large form of environmental manipulation because the size of the class, formal arrangements for instruction, supervision for times outside the room, and specific spatial and physical characteristics of the classroom are adjusted to allow learning to take place. For the child with multiple learning and behavior problems, such a class change is necessary. For the child with fewer problems who remains in the regular class, specific changes within the classroom and good cooperation between home and school are required, and a teacher aide may be needed. Ready availability of a special services staff person to provide support and specific suggestions is also important.

    Environmental manipulation in the home may mean giving the special child a room of his own, putting locks on siblings' and parents' doors, keeping valuables out of reach, and having concrete reminders of rules, such as charts, timers, or physical barriers.

    The brain dysfunction that causes a behavior disorder may have also caused some cognitive impairment or a learning disability. Learning difficulties must be carefully identified and given attention if management of an organic behavior disorder is to be effective. This is discussed in the next chapter.

NOTES

1. Boris Rubenstein, "Psychiatric Aspects of Chronic Handicaps" in *The Child with Disabling Illness: Principles of Rehabilitation,* 2nd ed., John A. Downey and Niels L. Low, eds. (New York: Raven Press, 1982) p. 566.

2. Salvador Minuchin and others, "A Conceptual Model of Psychosomatic Illness in Children" in *Annual Progress in Child Psychiatry and Child Development 1976.* (New York: Brunner/Mazel, 1977) pp. 319–340.

3. Rubenstein, "Psychiatric Aspects," p. 571.

4. Samuel Livingston, "Insight into the Personality of the Epileptic Youth," *Medical Insight,* August 1971, pp. 27 and 29.

5. William H. Olson and others, *Practical Neurology for the Primary Care Physician* (Springfield, IL: Charles C. Thomas, 1981) p. 167.

6. Georgia Travis, *Chronic Illness in Children: Its Impact on Child and Family.* (Stanford, CA: Stanford University Press, 1976) pp. 295–297.

6

ANALYZING THE BASIS OF A LEARNING PROBLEM AND FACILITATING LEARNING

> Milton was adamant. He shouted, "I'm NOT going to school!" His mother held her breath and counted to ten. This was the eighth confrontation she had had with her ten-year-old son in two weeks. It was always the same: "Why don't you want to go to school?" "It's too hard. The teacher says I'm lazy, that I could do the work if I'd try harder. But I *can't try any harder!*"

Milton needs more consideration than being told repeatedly by his mother that he must go to school even though it's hard. It is also irresponsible to tell a child he is lazy if his difficulty has not been investigated. There are many possible reasons for a learning problem in a child who has a chronic illness. For example, pain or anxious preoccupation can impair attention and concentration; sensory impairment, poor motor control or lethargy may be aspects of the illness or the side effects of medication; hyperactivity or poor memory functioning can result from medication; and interruptions in learning can result from missing school. Children with certain chronic disorders are overrepresented in the group having below-average mental ability. When illness or medical treatments involve the brain or central nervous system, there is a greater likelihood of mental retardation or learning disability. This chapter reviews the common components of a learning problem and the more specific factors relating to chronically ill children. Also, a step-by-step analysis of the basis of the problem is considered as the necessary precursor of successful remediation.

TEACHER FRUSTRATION

Teachers feel frustrated when they cannot keep all children up to level in their academic work. Indeed, they are often censured by the principal or criticized by the teacher of the next higher grade when a child's achievement levels are low. However, it is frequently impossible to keep a chronically ill child up to grade level in her work. This puts the teacher in a difficult position. The teacher is human and wants to be understanding and accepting of the child, but he is subject to many pressures. The teacher must not have unrealistic expectations of bringing an ill child up to grade level when it is impossible to do so; yet, he fears he will be subjected to criticism if he does not.

QUESTIONS TO ASK ABOUT THE CHILD'S CAPABILITIES

Children are born with an intrinsic drive to grow intellectually, to learn, to put their experiences to use. When a child is not learning at his age level, teachers should seek answers to the following questions:

1. Does the child have adequate vision and hearing?
2. Does the child have the mental ability for learning at an average rate?
3. Does the child have the requisite emotional maturity to get involved in academics, to pay attention in a group situation, and to work independently?
4. Does the child have the basic foundation of academic skills for the curriculum?
5. Is the child willing to put forth the effort needed to succeed?
6. Is the child's failure a result of emotional conflict?
7. Does the child have a learning disability?
8. Does the effect of medication the child is taking account for difficulties in mental functioning?
9. Does the child have enough physical and emotional energy to respond to learning tasks?

As most teachers know, a Child Study Evaluation provides answers to all of these questions at once. However, a Child Study Evaluation is usually available only for those children with the most complex problems or for those suspected of having a learning disability. In most cases, the teacher must make her own analysis of a learning problem. She should do this by systematically examining the most objective data she can gather, formulating a hypothesis regarding the basis of the problem, and testing the hypothesis by applying an appropriate strategy to remedy the problem. If the first hypothesis proves to be incorrect, the process should be repeated, using a new hypothesis.

DETERMINE SENSORY ADEQUACY

Determining whether or not a child has adequate vision and hearing is an easy task and is the place to begin when analyzing a learning problem. Visual and auditory screening should be readily available through the school nurse. Whether or not a child is suspected of having any difficulty seeing or hearing, these sensory functions should be tested. Children who are not paying attention may not be able to hear or see adequately, although the teacher may not think of this as a possible cause. Paradoxically, many children who show symptoms of visual difficulty (for example, a child who places a book close to his face, or a child who complains of blurriness after reading) prove not to have vision problems. These behaviors frequently reflect a child's psychological defenses. She hides herself by putting the book close to her face; she gets out of having to read more by saying her eyes have gotten blurry. Yet a teacher knows that a child's vision must be checked if she shows such obvious symptoms of visual difficulty.

A child who is passively resistant is often a master at acting as though he can't hear. Even if he obviously hears sometimes, the teacher will know to have his hearing checked. It is when children do not show any specific behavior that suggests a vision or hearing problem that teachers forget to have them checked. Teachers should remember that with some illnesses, vision or hearing changes can result from medical treatments or occur as complications of the illness. It is also possible that a chronically ill child, because of frequent absence, has missed the school's routine vision and hearing screening tests.

MEASURE MENTAL ABILITY

Chronically ill children in general can be expected to have an average or higher ability level. However, for children with cerebral palsy, spina bifida (myelomeningocele), Duchenne muscular dystrophy, and heart disease, the possibility of having below-average mental ability is fairly high. Approximately 75 percent of children with cerebral palsy have below-average mental abilities.[1] About 50 percent of children with spina bifida are below average,[2] and the rate is as high as 70 percent for the muscular dystrophy group as a whole.[3] Although the precise percentage is hard to establish, there is an increased incidence of low ability in children with heart disease, particularly those who were frequently cyanotic.[4] (Cyanosis is the lack of oxygenation of the blood and deprives the brain of adequate amounts of oxygen.)

Children who have been treated for cancer, with radiation to the head, may have lowered mental functioning.[5] Children who have sustained a high number of epileptic seizures also may suffer some degree of intellectual loss. Severe head injury and stroke can destroy brain cells, leading to cognitive impairment. In all of these instances, there are complex factors making it impossible to generalize or predict mental ability. The overall point is that lowered mental ability may often be found in children with a variety of chronic disorders.

A teacher should not assume that a child has below-average intelligence without having established this as a fact through individual testing. Many shy, passive, nonverbal children may seem dull and may actually be quite bright. The presence of a specific illness, or a facade of dullness, is not an accurate indicator of ability level. When there is a question in the teacher's mind about whether a child has adequate mental development for his age, she should first look in the child's cumulative folder to see if there is a record of group test results. If there are recent test results indicating average ability, she should feel reassured. However, if group test scores indicate a below-average ability level, she should have the validity of this checked against the findings of an individual test. Some children who score low on group tests actually have normal intelligence. If the child has an illness that is associated with a high incidence of below-average ability, an individual test of mental functioning should be recommended. The same is true if the child's illness has involved the brain in any way. An individual intelligence test is administered as part of a Child Study Evaluation (Chapter 12), but can also be done by any psychologist within or outside the school system.

Children with low mental ability are slow learners. In keeping with the bell-shaped curve concept, approximately one out of five children in regular classes would be slow learners if the child population were randomly distributed in all schools. Some of these children would be from the chronically ill group, but not all. However, children are not randomly distributed. We know that in some suburban areas, a select group of high-ability children are in attendance and, conversely, that a disproportionate number of low-ability children are found in poor and disadvantaged areas. A child of solid average ability can look like a slow learner in a suburban school where the pace of learning is geared to that of the majority of students who are above-average intellectually. On the other hand, where slow learners are the majority group, the pace of instruction is appropriately geared to the rate at which they can learn successfully. If a child is not learning satisfactorily and mental ability is a factor, the teacher must keep in mind the level of instruction she is using for the whole class.

Individualized Goals

For slow learners, and also for children with learning disabilities (to be discussed in a later section), the teacher should think about the psychological atmosphere of the classroom in regard to competition, the pace at which learning sequences should be presented, and the mode of instruction.

Children feel defeated or embarrassed within a highly competitive atmosphere if their abilities are well below the general level of the class. To maintain self-esteem, these children must learn to measure themselves and their progress in relation to an individualized set of goals. They must learn to compete with their own previous performance level rather than with the standard set for the majority of the class. All children are more comfortable by being challenged to improve their own performance rather than by trying to do as well or better than a classmate. This does not mean that the spirit of competition is eliminated. It just takes on a different emphasis—that of challenge—rather than of winning or being the best.

Pace Learning Sequences

Slow learners can master most of what is in the regular curriculum, but it takes them longer. In sequential learning, they need to master each step before going on to the next one. They require regular feedback to be sure they have understood correctly and to know if they are proceeding in the right way. This necessitates a great deal of supervision of the student's work efforts, much more than can be provided by the teacher. Use adult volunteers or peer tutors from the class to provide this kind of feedback and supervision.[6]

Peer Tutors

The most logical and readily available help for the slow student is a bright classmate. The bright students not only grasp the instruction easily, but they also finish their work quickly. The time they have to spare can be devoted to monitoring a slower classmate's work and offering help when needed. Both helper and helped will benefit from the relationship. Perhaps the child tutor can translate the conceptual ideas, even better than an adult, in such a way that they are understood by the slower student. This is because the peer shares the same "child level" way of thinking. Also, the positive feedback and encouragement a child receives from his same-age tutor may mean more to him than getting this kind of response from an adult. The child tutor feels gratified when his pupil does well. He is also likely to give support to his pupil on the playground, should he be teased or intimidated by other children.

I believe that the benefits for the bright child are equally great, possibly much more beneficial than pushing him intellectually. Peer tutoring makes the bright child feel important in nonacademic areas. It enhances his social consciousness, a most important attribute to encourage. Perhaps parents of gifted children would be less likely to focus only on their academic acceleration or enrichment if the school provided such significant experiences for developing them in broader ways.

In appointing a peer tutor, the teacher must convey a clear understanding of the regular, ongoing nature of the assignment and the responsibility involved. The child chosen by the teacher should be told that he can accept or decline the invitation to be a peer tutor. This should be done in a private conference. The teacher should tell the child that her relationship with the slow student will function somewhat like a buddy system. She will also be modeling for the class attitudes of helping and caring that the teacher wants all children to have. The teacher can point out that the slow learner will feel better about himself if he can do his work with less frustration and with less fear of failure. The slow child will also feel more secure, knowing that there is a friendly helper available, and he will be less worried. That will allow him to learn better.

Changes in Mode of Instruction

In addition to slowing down the pace of learning sequences, providing continual supervision, and giving regular feedback to the student, changes in the mode of instruction will be needed for the child with low mental ability. Instructional methods and techniques that do not rely heavily on verbal presentations are needed for the slower student. When giving instruction verbally, the teacher may also need to simplify the language level so that ideas are presented in clear, short statements.[7]

In order to make the effort to find a method of instruction that will be successful with slow learners, the teacher must believe that the student can learn the material. Experience and research have shown that when teachers expect students to be able to learn, they search for a method of instruction that works. The myth that slow learners just can't catch on is gradually disappearing, though it is still a common excuse for not trying alternative instructional modes.

It also helps if slow learners are a year older than their classmates. During the earliest school years, which concentrate on the very difficult task of learning to read, slow learners may develop a one-year lag in academic achievement that will be virtually impossible to make up. By seventh grade, a slow learner can be expected to show a two-year lag in achievement levels unless he has had the extra time and very specific help needed to keep up.

LOW MATURITY LEVEL

Children's behavioral maturity does not necessarily keep pace with their intellectual development. Many bright but immature children are mistakenly started in school too soon. Behaviors labeled as immature by teachers range from silly and inattentive to dependent, resistive, or lacking in initiative. Teachers frequently say, "He won't do anything unless I am standing right next to him" and protest, "He shouldn't be in this grade." However, it is too simplistic to believe that grade retention is the answer for all children displaying these behaviors.

Grade retention as a solution assumes that slow physical maturation accounts for the behavioral immaturity. This is not always a correct assumption. For example, it was not in Jerry's case.

> Jerry was retained in kindergarten because of immaturity, although he was five and one-half when he started school and physically large for his age. It was not until the end of first grade, after three years of failure, that he was diagnosed as having a severe learning disability. Precious time had been lost in getting appropriate educational help for him because it had been erroneously assumed that he just needed "more time to grow."

Immature behavior may be the expression of an emotional conflict or a defense for not being able to learn. For chronically ill children, the behavior may reflect confusion about independence and dependence and inhibition of initiative based on their medical experiences. The important issue regarding immaturity is deciding on the correct action to take. This requires an accurate assessment of the basis for the immaturity. Although grade retention is a beneficial solution for many, it is wise to base such a decision on the outcome of a Child Study Evaluation, or, at least, a psychological evaluation.

UNDERDEVELOPED SKILLS

When a child is failing tests and not completing work, first determine whether he has the requisite skills to do the work he is presented with. Can he read the words in his books? Can he understand them? If he is being taught multiplication, does he already know how to add and subtract?

The obvious is sometimes forgotten. The child who stares into space because he is too discouraged to do anything else may be dismissed as having an emotional problem, without the teacher's discovering that lack of skills is the cause of his lack of interest. When a child has missed a lot of school or has lacked the energy to respond to instruction over a period of time, it should be presumed that he may have skill deficits. A screening survey of basic skills does not take long to administer and should be given as a first step. If lags in achievement or gaps in specific skills are disclosed, curriculum materials can be adjusted, tutoring considered, and other adjustments made. Perhaps the results of the screening will indicate that a more complete assessment should be done, and a Child Study Evaluation can be arranged.

MOTIVATIONAL PROBLEMS

Aside from average mental ability, adequate behavioral maturity, and possession of appropriate skills, children must be willing to make the effort to learn. If a child is to be expected to put forth the necessary effort, she must believe that she has a chance to succeed. If she has experienced too much failure, she is likely to believe that she cannot succeed. "Why try?" she says to herself. "It won't do any good." If the atmosphere of the class is highly competitive and there are many bright students in the group, an average child might feel defeated before she even tries. She will say to herself, "There is no way I can win, be among the best, so what does it matter?"

There are also those children who want only to play or have fun. They have not learned to delay gratification, and any reward for working hard is too remote. When school tasks are fun, or easy, so that they can succeed quickly, these children are usually willing to do them, but not otherwise. Some children in the early grades need to be rewarded so they will make an effort. Other children have unmet social needs and want to use the classroom to obtain social gratification, rather than to do schoolwork. When any of these factors is operating, a child is considered to have a motivational problem.

When it has been determined that a child has the skills and abilities to do the work, the task is to entice him to do it. He may need to develop more self-confidence. If so, giving him short tasks in which he can expect to succeed—and telling him as soon as he has finishes that his work is correct—can help.

For the child who needs reward and gratification in the form of social approval and a pat on the back, working with an aide or volunteer on a one-to-one basis may increase his productivity. Behavior modification approaches (using charts, stars, special activity, and social rewards) may also prove successful with the child who needs rewards and who needs to learn to delay gratification.

Older children who are unmotivated may be bored or resistant to doing what an authoritarian person requires of them. Attempt to develop intrinsic motivation by making the learning project so attractive and satisfying that the child can't resist it. These children often rebel at school because they are not allowed sufficient autonomy at home. A need for some degree of self-determination may be the reason for their refusal to do schoolwork. Giving them some decision-making power with regard to learning tasks can prove to be motivating.

DEGREE OF EMOTIONAL CONFLICT

As children mature, they are faced with increasing demands for self-control, for delaying gratification, and for assuming responsibility. In school, a child must inhibit her wishes to play or be social, must sit still for long periods when she wishes for active movement, and must do the work assigned whether or not she wants to. Every child, in the normal course of growing up, experiences conflicts between doing what others want her to do and what she herself wishes to do. These normal conflicts must be mastered if normal social-emotional development is to take place.

Children also experience new and different fears as they grow to know more about the world. These fears must not be allowed to get out of proportion, and they too must be mastered. Cognitive development and school learning and productive use of fantasy help a child master these normal conflicts and fears. In the usual course of events, these normal emotional conflicts do not seriously interfere with learning. However, a child does require a normal expectable environment, one that is attuned to his developmental needs, if his built-in mechanisms for achieving mastery are to be effective. For a chronically ill child, the environment is often neither normal nor expectable; that is, the uncertainty of his illness precludes predicting what is going to happen to him, and when his usual routine includes frequent medical tests and treatments, visits to clinics or stays in the hospital, his environment is not the normal one of healthy children.

Children who have been, or are, chronically ill, have fears and conflicts that go beyond those that are considered normal. They also have less favorable environmental experiences. Thus, their opportunities for mastering normal fears and conflicts are reduced.

Emotional conflicts that interfere with learning are those normal ones that have not been mastered and also those extraordinary ones arising out of traumatizing experiences.

Conflicts that interfere with learning result from parental imperatives or inconsistent experiences in the environment that lead to mixed-up feelings about:

dependence — independence

good — bad

right — wrong

being adequate — being inadequate

being competent — being incompetent

When there are serious problems within the family, when the family has been disrupted by divorce or displaced by a recent move, or when a child's medical condition deteriorates, an ill child's normal emotional dilemmas will become compounded.

Children whose learning difficulties result primarily from an emotional problem need psychotherapy, either individual or family oriented. Their learning difficulties may clear up spontaneously as their emotional or family problems become resolved. However, concurrent tutoring by a warm and supportive teacher is a good idea. This is usually not provided by the school and should be arranged and paid for by the parents. If parents are unwilling or unable to provide psychological help for a child outside of school, the school's counseling services should be made available to facilitate some improvement in the child's performance.

LEARNING DISABILITY

Learning disability is another cause of failure to learn adequately or to keep up to grade level. The label *learning disability* has come into use during the last two decades, although children with learning disabilities existed long before the label was created. There have always been some children whose learning failure was inexplicable. These children did not have diagnosable emotional problems; they seemed to try and to *want* to learn, and they could see, hear, and understand. In fact, they appeared to be normal in every way except for their failure—or extreme difficulty—in learning to read, write, and spell, or, in some instances, to learn mathematics.

Confusion and Controversy

Psychologists and educators working in the area of learning disability *know* that it exists. However, confusion and controversy have accompanied the development of the study of learning disability. There are educators who insist that no such thing as learning disability exists. How can there be, they say, if learning disability cannot be defined? There has been much disappointment that a universally acceptable definition of learning disability has not been established. (The definition of learning disability contained in federal law is no longer acceptable to educational leaders.) Many professionals are concerned that far too many children are diagnosed as having a learning disability, and I agree. Developmental immaturity (starting a child in school before his cognitive, perceptual, speech, and behavior are sufficiently developed) is probably the basic problem with a high percentage of children who are diagnosed as having a learning disability.

There are many controversial issues, and the professional and political pressure groups continue to debate them.[8] There is no evidence of agreement on the horizon. As the professional leaders continue to disagree, it seems important to state my own position.

1. Although neither learning disabilities nor their causes are yet fully understood, there is abundant research and clinical evidence to substantiate that they do exist as a distinct entity.

2. The incidence of learning-disabled children has been grossly overestimated, probably because misdiagnosis is common. For every child with a learning disability, there are three more who have learning problems for a different reason.[9] Children most likely to be misdiagnosed as learning disabled are those who are developmentally immature.

3. When a definition is ultimately agreed upon, I believe it will state that differences in brain organization and brain function are the primary bases of learning disability. These differences in brain structure and function can occur through genetic transmission or from some exogenous factor. Exogenous events can occur before birth as a result of illness in the mother, medications taken by her, smoking, drinking, and so on. They can also occur as the result of prematurity, difficulties during delivery, or from a variety of later events. Insufficient oxygen to the brain, at birth, or during cyanotic episodes from any cause; traumatic head injury; viral illness involving the central nervous system; lead poisoning; stroke; endocrine disorders; postoperative brain tumor; and others are all events that can cause alterations in brain function. A variety of medications are also known to alter brain function.

4. When the confusion has cleared away and developmental immaturity dealt with by delaying school entrance or by grade retention, it should be possible to establish diagnostic criteria to be adhered to by those entrusted to diagnose learning disability. Diagnostic instruments are being improved and refined, and these will make it possible to demonstrate that deviations in brain organization and function exist. Diagnosticians will be required to have expertise in neuropsychology, as well as in clinical psychology, and in the psychology of learning. Diagnosis will depend on clinical judgment, the results of tests, and the history either of early learning failure in a close relative (genetic transmission) or of an exogenous event that could have altered brain function.

5. When learning disabilities are more fully understood, three general subgroupings will emerge:

   a. Children who, although developmentally mature and of normal intelligence, have serious difficulty acquiring the basic skills of reading, spelling, writing, or mathematics. These children will be identified during their earliest school years.

   b. Children who have a lot of difficulty organizing and relating ideas and information. They will have trouble generalizing and transferring learning; that is, applying learned information in new situations. These children will acquire the basic skills at a normal rate. Their problems will probably not become clearly evident until eight, nine, or ten years of age.

c. Children who have difficulty learning in a large group situation, when the instructional level has become fairly complex. These are children who have language difficulties or difficulties focusing attention on relevant aspects, or difficulty retaining directions, or difficulty with the comprehension or memory of oral instruction. This latter occurs either because material is presented too fast or is not well-ordered, or the mode of presentation is too complex or abstract. These children's problems may not become apparent until fourth grade or later. The reason for this perhaps is because the teacher has intuitively adapted to the younger child's instructional needs and has also offered a lot of extra help to the child during the early stages of academic learning. The younger child may also have felt freer to ask for additional explanations than the older child does.

The School's Role

A child with a learning disability needs specialized help from an educational specialist. The educational specialist, usually called *a Learning Disabilities teacher,* has been trained in techniques that can be effective with the learning-disabled child. He usually works with a child on a one-to-one basis, but occasionally in a small group of two or three. Specialized individual help should be available in the school, at no extra cost to parents, once a child has been diagnosed as having a learning disability.

A child may have been diagnosed as having a learning disability and yet may not require specialized help. He will need help if he has a lag in academic skills. However, some bright and motivated students with other kinds of learning disability discover their own strategies of compensating. Children with these kinds of disability who do need help are *taught* compensatory strategies.

It is sometimes difficult to distinguish between learning disabilities and developmental immaturity and emotionally based learning problems. The educational symptoms may be similar for each group. Children who have a learning disability are usually frustrated and upset because they cannot meet academic expectations. They are relieved when their problem is discovered and are usually eager to accept tutoring. On the other hand, emotionally based learning problems are commonly rooted in conflict, anger, and rebellion. Children who are passively resistant, anxious, and depressed also have learning problems. These children often resist tutoring. If an incorrect diagnosis of the basis of a learning problem has been made, the child's reaction to tutoring may be the clue indicating the diagnosis should be questioned.

How Medical Treatments Affect Energy Levels

When medical treatment or surgery lead to permanent changes in brain function, a learning disability is likely to result. Other medical treatment, such as certain drugs prescribed for epilepsy, intractable asthma, and severe juvenile rheumatoid arthritis, may cause transitory alterations in brain processes. These children encounter interference with learning because of the fluctuations in their ability to attend, respond, and do work, caused by the effects of their medications. Some medications cause a child to be hyperreactive to stimuli, as well as hyperactive. Other medications have the opposite effect, causing a child to be dull, lethargic, or drowsy. The hyperstimulated child will have trouble sitting still and keeping his attention focused. On the other hand, the child who is lethargic or drowsy will be lacking in energy. Her ability to attend and respond will be markedly reduced. Medications that alter the energy level and degree of responsiveness in either direction will cause a child to experience decreased learning efficiency. Whenever it is suspected that a child's medication is affecting his learning, the teacher should consult with the child's doctor.

GRADE RETENTION

If a chronically ill child is absent for most or all of a school year and has been too ill to do much schoolwork, the possibility of grade retention must be considered. I have also previously mentioned that grade retention can be a partial solution for children who are slow learners. It is frequently indicated for children who start school before they are developmentally ready. Some children with learning disabilities may also benefit from grade retention as a part of an overall plan.

Staying back in a grade has significant ramifications for a child and his family, and the decision to do this must be cautiously and carefully considered. Ideally, the decision should be based on the results of a complete psychological and educational evaluation, but this is not always possible. When the decision must be based on information other than a recent individual evaluation, the following criteria should be considered:

- Young age; enrollment in kindergarten was before age five for girls, age five and one-half for boys
- Social and behavioral difficulties
- Resistance to doing work based on a feeling of being pressured
- Academic lag of significant degree
- Small physical size and/or motor immaturities (not including motor problems resulting from cerebral palsy or other handicapping conditions)
- Low-average or below-average IQ
- Both parents in agreement with the retention

At least five of these seven criteria should be present to validate grade retention. Some young children do well in school. Some slow learners would not have to be retained if they had been older when they started school.

Reactions to Retention and How to Guide Parents

A child invariably feels that she is a failure and a big disappointment to her mother and father if she must repeat a grade. Parents frequently perceive their child's need to be retained as a blow to the family's esteem. They become anxious about whether the retention will really help and whether their child will have to face difficulty and frustration with learning throughout her school years. They worry about their child's being teased and taunted for having failed. If either parent has a bad memory of his or her own retention, these worries will be magnified.

As the parents take a central role in helping their child accept retention and in teaching him how to deal with any negative feedback he gets from others, it is imperative that they be in agreement with a planned retention. Parents will need guidance in how to turn the potentially negative experience of retention into an opportunity for growth.

A small but very important book is now available that tells how to help a child when a decision has been made by the teacher and the parents that he must repeat a grade. The book is called *Staying Back*. It presents children's stories in their own words of their school experiences before and after staying back. Illustrated stories of children who were retained in grades one through six are presented. The stories are appropriate for reading to or being read by children. The authors provide lists of questions that can be put to children to open a discussion and talk about feelings. Although the stories are intended for use with the child who is to be held back, I believe teachers could make all children sensitive to the issue if they incorporated the stories and discussions into the regular curriculum. I think this book is so unique and valuable that it should be in every school and public library.

The following material is adapted from Dr. Barry Dym's message to parents contained in *Staying Back*. Dr. Dym offers seven steps to be followed in helping the child who must repeat a grade.* He advises:

Step One: Let your child know you love him or her.

Step Two: Listen. Before offering reassurances or suggestions, let your child talk freely and express as much or as little of his feelings as he can or wishes to share.

Step Three: Try to identify exactly what staying back means to your child. How does he see himself? This will give you the information you need to help turn the disappointment around into something positive.

Step Four: Explore what your child's staying back means to you and to other family members.

Step Five: Using your child's own ideas, "reframe" the experience of being kept back as an opportunity to succeed. For example, it may be a chance to stop struggling on the bottom rung of the class.

Step Six: While letting your child "off the hook" of failure, you still need to state firm, clear expectations about hard work for greater success in the future.

Step Seven: Find some ways to pay special attention to the things your child does well.

Dr. Dym discusses each step so that what is to be done is clearly understood. Teachers could memorize the steps, as a sort of litany, in order to advise parents when retention is decided upon. Having the book available to lend to parents is even better. Ask the principal or the PTA to get several copies to be shared by all teachers and for lending to parents.

---

*Janice Hobby and Gabrielle and Daniel Rubin, *Staying Back*, with a message for parents by Barry M. Dym, Ph.D., published by Triad Publishing, Gainesville, FL, © 1982. Used by permission.

Catching Up with the Class

If a child is a known slow learner, I would caution teachers not to tell the parents or the child that he will no longer be at the bottom of the class after repeating. Many slow learners will still be at the bottom of the class, and they will always have to work very hard. However, as they improve their skills and gain maturity, they should be able to persevere in their schoolwork with less of a sense of frustration. Slow learners should be told that retention will give them an opportunity to catch up with the class. They usually know they are quite far behind.

NOTES

1. Eugene E. Bleck, "Cerebral Palsy" in *Physically Handicapped Children: A Medical Atlas for Teachers,* 2nd ed., Eugene E. Bleck and Donald A. Nagel, eds. (New York: Grune and Statton, 1982) p. 72.

2. Georgia Travis, *Chronic Illness in Children: Its Impact on Child and Family.* (Stanford, CA: Stanford University Press, 1976) p. 458.

3. Eugene E. Bleck, "Muscular Dystrophy" in Bleck and Nagel, *Medical Atlas,* p. 391.

4. Travis, *Chronic Illness,* p. 264.

5. Gerald P. Koocher and John E. O'Malley, *The Damocles Syndrome: Psychosocial Consequences of Surviving Childhood Cancer.* (New York: McGraw-Hill, 1981) p. 164.

6. Benjamin Bloom, *All Our Children Learning* (New York: McGraw-Hill, 1980) pp. 139–142.

7. Ibid. pp. 161–163.

8. "L. D. Definition," Feature series of articles in *Journal of Learning Disabilities,* Vol. 16, No. 1, January 1983, pp. 6–31.

9. Robert H. Bruininks, Gertrude M. Glaman, and Charlotte R. Clark, *Prevalence of Learning Disabilities: Findings, Issues, and Recommendations.* Research Report No. 20, Department of Health, Education, and Welfare, U.S. Office of Education, Bureau of Education for the Handicapped, June 1971, p. 5.

7

Helping a Child Prepare for Hospitalization and Making the Transition Back to School

The news was bad. Mother and the doctor were discussing another operation. Lynn knew she would have to be brave like the last time. She also knew that she wasn't going to believe that malarky about the "good" things she heard before, meant to keep her from being upset about being in the hospital. She had learned that operations are very scary no matter how many reassuring things you are told or how many pretend shots you give the teddy bear. It did help though, to have lots of people she knew put on surgical masks, she decided. "When you get used to your family and friends having only eyes," she reminded herself, "you can feel better in the operating room because you're less afraid of all those strange faceless eyes that come at you there."

Hospitalization is a common experience for chronically ill children, although modern pediatric practice discourages it except when absolutely necessary. This chapter discusses what constitutes adequate preparation for hospitalization and the teacher's role in regard to the hospital experience.

FROM SCHOOL TO HOSPITAL: THE TRANSITION

When a child leaves school to enter a hospital, he experiences a major transformation in his world. School is a place where sights and sounds are colorful and lively. Faces are alert, curious, smiling, or expectant, and there is a kaleidoscope of activity. In the hospital, people move slowly. Faces wear frowns and grimaces. Some people can't walk and are pushed in wheelchairs or are flat on their backs on tables with wheels. The atmosphere is quiet, and a sense of dread pervades. Gray cement walls open upon eerie-looking machines and unfamiliar equipment, while people in crisp white clothes hurry about with a sense of urgency and efficiency.

When anticipating hospitalization, children typically have scary thoughts and fantasies, based on insufficient or incorrect information. It is important for them to verbalize their fantasies so adults can correct any misinformation and help reduce fears. Children also need a lot of reassurance. They want to know where a parent will be at all times and when they can expect a parent to be with them. They need to know that there will be discomfort and pain and that it is all right to cry and to feel angry about the things to which they must submit.[1]

School-age children may have experienced hospitalization during their preschool years. Depending on the nature of their previous hospital experience, they may have only a moderate degree of anxiety about a subsequent hospitalization. If a child has had a favorable experience, he will be familiar with what to expect, knowing that his needs will be met and that he will receive support from parents and hospital staff. However, school-age children almost always have some anticipatory anxiety when they know they must be hospitalized. They worry about the procedures they must undergo. They think about the pain they must endure and wonder if this means their illness is getting worse. They worry about getting behind in schoolwork and begin to think about all they will be missing while they are gone. They fear they will be forgotten by friends.[2]

If a school-age child has never been hospitalized or has had an unfavorable experience in a hospital, her anxiety may be unusually high. She may suddenly be unable to function in school or may not want to go to school.

THE TEACHER'S ROLE

The teacher should be informed as soon as a parent knows of an impending hospitalization. If a chronically ill child shows signs of increased anxiety, the teacher should call the parents to ask what the cause might be. Perhaps the child will have told the teacher she is to be hospitalized because she feels free to express her worries at school.

The teacher should call the parents to discuss the impending hospitalization when he learns about it from the child, realizing that parents might have neglected to inform him because of *their* anxiety or because they are not sophisticated enough to know that they should inform the school. These parents may also know little about preparing for the hospitalization, which includes making arrangements for a home or hospital teacher through the district office.

A child can be helped to deal with anxiety about impending hospitalization in a number of ways. Parents have the major responsibility for doing this, but teachers can also be helpful, particularly in guiding parents. Teachers must be aware that a child may express fears and worries while in school and be prepared to respond. The best way to respond is to ask questions. Questions are a way to find out more clearly what the child is worried about, and they also serve to help him think for himself—find ways to reassure himself or to realize he can and should ask parents to answer some of his questions. Children come to teachers for answers when they perceive their parents as anxious, preoccupied, or emotionally distant. The teacher should remind himself that the primary responsibility for preparing a child for hospitalization belongs to the parents.

The Teacher as Liaison

The teacher can act as a go-between for the child, making it possible for him to talk with his parents. To do this, the teacher should call the parents in for a conference and, with the child present, help the child talk to them. At the same time, the teacher can learn such important things as where he will be hospitalized, for how long, whether the hospital has a preparation program, a child-life program, a schoolroom, and so forth. If the parent does not know the answers to some of these questions, the teacher will be implying that the parent should get the answers.

In some instances, when a teacher acts as liaison between a child and the family, she speaks for him. She tells the parent what she has learned directly from the child, checking back with him from time to time to find out if she is stating his concerns correctly. This procedure is necessary for younger children and for older children who are shy. With a child who is less shy, the teacher may need only to get him started talking to his parent and then give encouragement along the way. The teacher should always start by inviting the child to speak for himself but be ready to speak for him if he cannot. The teacher may also need to tell the parent how to prepare and reassure the child about the impending hospitalization.

Guiding the Family

Preparing a child for hospitalization means telling him what to expect regarding routines and rules while there and about what is going to happen medically. Being in the hospital means being separated from parents, siblings, and friends. It means being with strangers in an unfamiliar place. It means being pushed and rolled and poked and thumped by these strangers. Invasive procedures such as suppositories and enemas may be encountered for the first time.

Reading a child books and stories about hospitalization, about children being separated from parents, and about children dealing with their fears can help a child prepare for hospitalization. A teacher who reads to her class regularly may choose such a story when she knows that one of her pupils is to be hospitalized. This will help the child share his anticipatory anxiety and give his classmates a chance to be empathic. She can also give parents the names of appropriate books.

Many hospitals have preadmission preparation programs for the child and the family. Such programs may present a slide show depicting a child entering the hospital and all the things that happen to him there. Then the presenter will typically engage in a discussion with the children aimed at eliciting questions, feelings, and fears. The presenter, who is likely to be the child-life worker from the pediatric unit, may engage in medical play with the children. Medical objects such as stethoscopes, blood pressure cuffs, shot syringes, and masks will be used, with the aim of alleviating the child's fears. He may be given a coloring book of hospital things and a throwaway syringe and paper objects to take home.[3] If such a program is available, the parents' job of preparing a child for hospitalization will be easier. The teacher should encourage the child's parents to have him participate in any preadmission program that is available.

Allaying the Child's Fears about Falling Behind in School

The teacher can give the child direct help in dealing with his concerns about falling behind in schoolwork and being away from his classmates. She can make sure he has an educational instructor while he is in the hospital and at home afterward. Large general hospitals and children's hospitals usually have a schoolroom and teachers on staff, but in other situations, the local school district must send a tutor for the hospitalized child. The classroom teacher should advise a parent to arrange in advance for a tutor to come to the hospital. She should also see that the tutor works on appropriate lessons with the child.

IN THE HOSPITAL

Hospitalization for children is potentially traumatic. Recognition of this fact led to the formation of the Association for the Care of Children's Health (ACCH) in 1965. This organization is dedicated to helping children and their families cope in health care settings. Through the efforts and actions of its members, much progress has been made in humanizing the hospital experience for children. The standards set by ACCH for hospitals having a pediatric unit include a preadmission preparation program for the child and the family; twenty-four-hour visiting for parents, as well as having rooming-in arrangements and allowing parents to help care for their child; child-life program and hospital school program. ACCH also advocates that the child and the family should receive educational and emotional support before, during, and after medical and surgical procedures, and that they should have help in planning for the return to home and school.[4]

A large number of hospitals have responded to these recommendations by liberalizing parents' visits and allowing parents of young children to stay around the clock. Hospitals now more commonly provide a playroom, schoolroom, and child-life program. However, there are still many hospitalized children who do not have access to these extremely important necessities.

When a hospital provides a child-life program and preparation for medical procedures, traumatization from the hospital experience will be reduced. There is the added possibility that the hospital experience may have a positive impact on psychological growth. Inasmuch as a child learns to master a very difficult experience, she will be prepared to cope with future stresses. Given the proper help, she can understand, integrate, and master the fear created by the threatening things that happen to her in the hospital. She may then be able to generalize her experience for mastering other frightening situations encountered later.[5]

The Role of the Child-Life Worker

The child-life specialist is a person trained in child development. Coming from many different professional backgrounds—psychology, education, and nursing to mention a few—the child-life worker is specially trained to work with sick children. She oversees children's psychological well-being while they are hospitalized. Using play therapy techniques, the child-life specialist prepares a child for surgery and helps him master the anxieties that still persist afterward. (This might also be done by a nurse or resident doctor.) She plans play, social, and educational programs that nourish and enrich him. Once or twice a week, the worker holds a group therapy play session, sometimes called *medical play*. The children are encouraged to project their experiences and feelings in play. Children in the four to seven age group often have intense rage about the things that have been done to them. They are prone to outbursts and uncooperative behavior. Through play they learn to master their rage and usually become more cooperative. All children become more accepting of what happens to them as a result of the medical play therapy.[6]

The planned projects can help children maintain their sense of self-worth and address their feelings of isolation from familiar peers. For example, one project involved having children write stories and draw pictures about their particular illness or injury and what they had gone through. These were collected, put into magazine form each week, and copied for distribution to family and friends.

The child-life worker is available for support to both child and parents. She may have a supply of games and toys that can be borrowed by parents or other visitors to use in play with the ill child. Books that can help a child deal with the hospital experience or help the parent deal with special issues may also be available for borrowing.

The child-life worker is each child's special person while he is hospitalized. She is the liaison between him and other workers and services in the hospital. She may brief a home or hospital tutor about his needs and interests and about his illness. She may talk to a physical or occupational therapist about feelings that he could not express directly to them. She may alert the pediatric social worker that the family may be in need of services. She also helps the child keep in contact with the school and his friends. She may transmit messages by phone to his teacher or help him write or call a friend.[7]

PROVIDING CONTINUITY OF EDUCATION

If children are to continue their academic learning while hospitalized, they need a quiet place removed from "sick" and "play areas" where instruction can be given. The room should resemble a schoolroom; there should be desks and a chalkboard. It is beneficial for children to be involved with schoolwork while they are hospitalized. It not only gives them continuity in their learning, but it also brings a sense of normalcy to the daily routine. Becoming absorbed in thoughts and ideas beyond illness and confinement is good for their mental health.

Even if the hospital provides a school program, the regular class-room teacher should be involved, to be sure that the child is getting similar instruction to what he would be receiving in class at his own school. If the teacher does not receive a call from the hospital teacher, she should take the initiative in making the call herself. The parents will probably need to pick up the child's books, unless he took them with him in the first place.

KEEPING THE CLASSMATES IN TOUCH WITH THE HOSPITALIZED CHILD

If it is possible and the teacher has the time, she may wish to visit the child while he is hospitalized. This frequently is neither reasonable nor feasible, and no teacher should cause herself hardship to do this. It is important, though, to communicate with the ill child by sending periodic messages about what is happening at school. The teacher may send messages to the child via parent, hospital tutor, or child-life worker. Classmates should be encouraged to send cards or letters.

Teachers often have card- or letter-writing as a class project, with all pupils doing this at the same time. When the hospital stay is short, the sick child may enjoy receiving twenty or thirty cards all at once. However, if a child is to be hospitalized for two weeks or longer, getting a few cards every few days will be more satisfying. The teacher can organize the card-sending activity to last for the duration of the child's hospital stay. Have classmates take turns, one or two children writing on subsequent days or weeks. This will work best if the class receives news of the sick child.

If the hospitalized child is not too ill to write or draw, he should respond to his classmates' messages directly by telling them what is happening to him in the hospital. It is difficult for class members to feel in contact or to know whether their efforts are appreciated unless there is response from the other end. Young children who cannot write can draw pictures or create cards by cutting and pasting. Both the schoolmate and the sick child can feel in contact when receiving a message, whether verbal or pictorial, which is on his own level of ability. If continuity of interest and caring is maintained between the sick child and his classmates, his return to school will be easier.

PREPARING FOR THE RETURN TO SCHOOL

A child should never go directly from the hospital back to school unless the hospitalization has been brief and the child has not become anxious and upset by being away from home. A child who has been hospitalized for tests to adjust or evaluate medication or to stabilize physiology during an acute episode of the illness may not be particularly upset by his hospital experience. When he has had several short hospitalizations of this kind, he knows what to expect, and if he has an adaptable temperament, the experience will most likely be perceived as a routine part of his life.

More frequently, a child's hospital experience isolates and humiliates him. He must relinquish his autonomy, accept the rigidity of hospital routines, and adapt to frequent changes in caretakers. These adjustments will be most difficult for the child who is slow to warm up or who is timid and very uncomfortable in unfamiliar surroundings. If a child has a negative temperament (and seven to ten percent of children do) he will have difficulty eliciting comforting responses from his caretakers. Sometimes children get the idea that their chances of getting better depend on strict adherence to hospital rules and rituals. These children will experience anxiety when they return home to different routines and a less predictable order to their day.

A child's transition back to family life and to a schedule that includes going to school will take time and effort. When he is sufficiently improved to return home, he must begin to re-channel his thoughts, concerns, and psychic energy. While in the hospital, his major concern has been his illness and his physical body. His energy has been consumed with physical survival. Now everyone thinks he is well enough to go back to school. It is too much to expect that a child can make the transition from the culture of the hospital, where he was required to be a submissive, dependent creature, to the culture of the school, where he will be expected to assume initiative and to act independently, without being given time, preparation, and assurance of support.

In returning home, an ill child may find that there is emotional distance between him and his family; they feel like strangers to each other. They will need time to rediscover a sense of intimacy with each other, and the ill child will need time to regain his sense of belonging.

The Trauma of Having "Changed"

Children who have experienced any change in their appearance will be very apprehensive about returning to school. The changes may be slight or temporary—for example, minor scars, or baldness caused by cancer treatment. The changes may be major—for example, losing a limb through amputation, having large scars in obvious places, or being confined to a wheelchair.

Children who have been hospitalized because they have suffered head injury or other illnesses that involved the brain may be different than they were before for other than physical reasons. These children may behave differently and may no longer be the excellent students they previously were. Changes in behavior and learning will be difficult for the teacher and a child's peers to understand and accept. It is possible that these children may no longer be able to manage in a regular class. Thoughtful preplanning for return to school is necessary for such children, and teachers or principals will need to caution parents about this.

Children's worries about returning to school center around the fear that they won't be recognized if their body or appearance has changed, fear that they won't be able to do the work, and fear that classmates will reject or exclude them.

If a child's appearance has changed markedly while he has been hospitalized, the teacher should ask the parent to send recent pictures of him to school before he reenters. The teacher and classmates will have a chance to get used to him as he now appears. This kind of prior conditioning should reduce surprised or startled reactions that would upset the returning child.

Helping the Child Fit In

If the child reenters school at the beginning of the fall term, special concerns about his becoming part of the class are not as necessary. But when he enters a class that is already established, his problem is different.

When a class becomes a cohesive whole, it takes on group properties. Rules govern its operation: rules made by the teacher that are explicit, and rules that are implicit in the relationships among the group members. There is an unspoken leader among the children, and a hierarchical organization, determined by the intellectual, social, and physical skills of the group members.

A child who comes into an already functioning class is a stranger entering a closely knit group, whether or not he already knows or is friends with individual members of the class. He must find a niche for himself within the already formed organization, and this is not an easy task. He must first deduce how the group functions and what the position and role of each classmate is, whether he be misfit, loner, or group leader. If he already knows some of the children, he can use their help in gaining a place for himself in the group. The teacher, keeping an alert eye on transactions among the children, may be able to facilitate the child's efforts to get a feeling of belonging.

With awareness of these factors, the teacher and the parent can avoid giving the reentering child false reassurance. An apprehensive child entering an already formed group is usually reminded of the children in the class he already knows. He should also be told that it will be hard to get into the swing of things coming back into the class at this time. Acknowledged understanding by the teacher and the parent that it is hard to come into an already formed class group will be helpful to the returning child.

PREPARING THE CLASS FOR THE CHILD'S RETURN

The teacher can prepare the class by announcing that the child is expected to return to school and by asking the class to plan how they can make him feel welcome. The more the class knows of his experience in the hospital and what his worries and fears are about returning to school, the more empathetic they can feel and act toward him. If there is no way to know these factors, if the child is new to the school, or if his parents have not told the teacher anything, the children should be asked to imagine what he experienced in the hospital and what he might be feeling about returning to school.

The idea that the previously hospitalized child might have difficulty relating to children in the class should be brought up during the planning. The ill child's sense of isolation, the fact that he and his family have been scared and worried, and the idea that he might not have had a chance to learn some of the games every child takes for granted should be mentioned. The class should be told that the child could be shy or belligerent, easily hurt, or likely to think others do not like him, and that many chronically ill children have these feelings. The class member who makes a friendly gesture to the new child should be forewarned not to be hurt or concerned if his overture is rebuffed. The ill child may have to test whether people really care, by seeing if they will still accept him even if he reacts negatively.

PREPARING THE CLASS FOR THE IMMINENT DEATH OF A CLASSMATE

When a child has a very serious illness, he may continue to attend school while his condition is worsening. There comes a time when the classmates realize that the next departure for the hospital means their friend will die. Hope is maintained to the end, and both the parents and the child may engage in a practice known as *mutual pretense* in order to deny their knowledge of imminent death.

As a part of this well-developed ritual, children may want to take their schoolbooks to the hospital. Acting as if they intend to study means they expect to go on living. Teachers should participate in this pretending ritual by giving the child an assignment if he should ask for it.

With our present knowledge about how to help children understand death and to deal with their anxiety and grief about it, a classmate's death can be a learning experience.

The mother or father of a child who dies can be invited to come and talk to the class. Not all parents will feel able or willing to talk to the class, but the teacher should extend the invitation. Parents who have been willing to do this have found it a rewarding experience. Helping their child's friends deal with the loss enables the parents to work through their own grief. In one such instance, the best friend of a child who died wanted to know if it was all right to give away a favorite T-shirt that was identical to the one her dead friend had had. The mother assured her that this was a natural reaction and that she most surely should do just that, if she wanted to.

ACKNOWLEDGING THE CLASSMATES' GRIEF

When a child dies, the whole class and perhaps most of the school will be affected. In their book, *They Need to Know: How to Teach Children about Death,** Audrey K. Gordon and Dennis Klass indicate that it is important to have some kind of ceremony so that the death can be publicly acknowledged and children can have a communal expression of grief. The child's teacher should take the initiative in planning this with the principal. If the child is not well known outside his own class, the acknowledgment and communal expression of grief may be simply a schoolwide announcement (possibly over the intercom) followed by a period of silence. Then, within the dead child's classroom, a more extended period can be devoted to remembering him, reading poetry, or listening to music.

Gordon and Klass suggest that the teacher tell the students (if they are old enough) the visiting hours at the funeral home and possibly give a lesson on funeral etiquette. Students should be given an

---

*Adapted from *They Need to Know* by Audrey K. Gordon and Dennis Klass, © 1979 by Prentice-Hall, published by Prentice-Hall, Englewood Cliffs, NJ 07632.

address to which personal sympathy notes can be sent. If the teacher plans a condolence call, she may wish to invite students who want to, to accompany her. She should allow groups of students who feel the need to plan and execute more concrete forms of expressing condolence or acts of commemoration.

The death of an ill child will be profoundly felt by his surviving siblings. Healthy siblings face many difficulties arising from the family stress when there is a chronically ill child in the home. The next chapter will discuss the variety of ways that siblings are affected.

NOTES

1. *A Child Goes to the Hospital* and *Preparing Your Child for Repeated or Extended Hospitalization* (Pamphlets) (Washington, DC: Association for the Care of Children's Health, 1981, 1982).

2. Ibid.

3. Interview with Sorrell Stanton, child-life specialist, Evanston Hospital, Evanston, IL, Spring 1983.

4. *Your Hospital: Meeting the Special Needs of Children* (Pamphlet) (Washington, DC: Association for the Care of Children's Health, 1981).

5. Susan Droske and Sally Francis, *Pediatric Diagnostic Procedures*. (New York: John Wiley and Sons, 1981) p. 4.

6. Mary Ann Adams, "A Hospital Play Program, Helping Children with Serious Illness." *American Journal of Orthopsychiatry*, 46 (3): 416–424, 1976, p. 421.

7. Sorrell Stanton (Interview).

8

HELPING HEALTHY
SIBLINGS
IN SCHOOL

"My parents must be crazy," Jeff told himself. "Why are they taking me to that hospital learning clinic for tests? Rudy's the one who needs tests. All the time in school I keep thinking of ways to get rid of Rudy, or at least get him a new brain. He's the cause of all my problems. It's a mystery to me why he's had all those operations and is in a special class. But geez, he breaks my toys, keeps me up all night with his nightmares, and even wets his pants, and my parents don't do a thing about it!"

Healthy siblings often present a wide range of symptoms in school, from physical complaints to learning problems. The symptoms are the child's message that he is upset or has unmet needs or can't share his feelings. The child communicates through symptoms because he doesn't feel free to use more direct methods. Experience indicates that healthy siblings are wondering "What is wrong with my brother or sister?" They are often panicked by their concerns but afraid to ask questions. Sometimes they can't ask because they feel left out by the family.

Interestingly, siblings' symptoms may only emerge in school. At home, siblings usually valiantly try to reduce family stress by taking on responsibilities beyond their years, controlling their emotions in adult fashion, and accepting restrictions on their freedom and autonomy. They try very hard to be good, so they won't add to the family burden they so accurately perceive. If the family's stress is exacerbated by parental divorce or separation, the healthy child's efforts will be increased. The child who is irresponsible about his work at school may be overly responsible at home. A teacher should not assume that a child who is irresponsible at school is also irresponsible at home, particularly when it is known that he has a chronically ill or disabled sibling. His irresponsibility at school is often a reaction to having to be too adultlike at home. His irresponsibility is his way of saying that he is still a child and needs to be taken care of.

SIBLINGS' NEED FOR INFORMATION

In their effort to protect the healthy children from distressing facts, or simply because they are too busy and preoccupied, parents frequently do not give the other children in the family enough information about the illness. They may believe that the children are not capable of understanding. They may not realize that a sibling who was too young to understand when the illness was first diagnosed is now old enough to be told. They may assume that the child knows what they know, without ever having been given information. They may be afraid that the sibling will tell the ill child things they feel he should not know. For whatever reason, it is clear that many siblings do not know what is wrong with their brother or sister. In the case of childhood cancer, one study showed that almost one-fourth of the boys and girls did not know their siblings had cancer.[1] Most had a poor understanding of their sibling's illness. They were not aware, for example, that the illness was life-threatening.

SIBLINGS' GUILT ABOUT THE ILLNESS

Sisters or brothers may feel guilty because they imagine they have caused or brought on the illness through something they did or failed to do.

Jennifer was such a child.

> Ten-year-old Jennifer has asthma, but her attacks are infrequent, and she and her family take them in stride. Younger brother Paul had always been a concern to the parents. Since birth, he had a variety of medical and developmental difficulties that created severe anxiety for the parents. Now, at age six, Paul also developed asthma. Jennifer is sure she has given it to him and feels very guilty and upset. For the first time in her school career, she has started doing poorly.

Siblings also may feel guilty when they have negative or angry feelings toward the ill sibling. They often harbor a fear of contracting the same disorder. These feelings and fears can usually be relieved by giving the child accurate information and reassurance. The teacher should consult with the parents about this.

SIBLINGS' NEED TO SHARE FEELINGS

When siblings do know and understand how serious and life-threatening an illness is, they may feel anxious, upset, and sad, as do their parents. But if parents do not want to see that their healthy children are anxious and worried, these children cannot share their sad feelings with the parents. They may begin to feel shut out from their parents' emotional field. If there are several siblings, all older than the sick child, they may draw together and try to nurture and reassure each other. They can share feelings of resentment, anger, and anxiety with each other, along with their sadness and fears. By such sharing, the intensity of their anxious feelings can be reduced to a more bearable level.

Jealousy of the ill child is experienced by many healthy siblings, although this is not as prevalent as some think. In those who experience jealousy, it is a case of normal sibling rivalry becoming exacerbated by the obvious special considerations extended to the ill child by the parents.

Parents change in their behavior toward the ill child once a serious or life-threatening illness is diagnosed. This has been substantiated repeatedly by researchers and is an understandable occurrence. Most apparent is the fact that they no longer require the sick child to live up to the behavioral standards of their healthy children. For example, eight-year-old Sarah could not understand why her sick sister was not required to share her toys, as everyone else in the family was expected to. Others cannot see why the sick sibling gets away with doing no chores, or that he is the one who usually gets to decide what TV programs will be watched.

Although jealousy on the part of the healthy sibling is easily understandable to an outsider, the family may reproach him for it. Made to feel ashamed for feeling this way, the healthy brother or sister may learn to repress or displace the jealousy. When a healthy sibling is having jealousy problems with peers in school or is jealous of the teacher's attention to other children, the problem may stem from jealousy toward the ill sibling that cannot be expressed directly.

PSEUDO-ADULTHOOD AND UNFULFILLED NEEDS

Having a sick sibling may thrust a boy or girl into pseudo-adulthood. Parents frequently must delegate caretaking responsibilities to the healthy child. The healthy sibling may also need to take on many household chores as well. These may include, for the older school-age child, cooking and cleaning jobs and may extend to responsibilities toward the sick child as well as younger siblings. The financial burden placed on the family by the sick child's medical and special equipment bills may make it necessary for both parents to work full time. The children shoulder their share of the burden by becoming responsible beyond their years. Those who are not given adult responsibilities within the home may be expected to find ways to earn money outside the home.

Children who must take on adult responsibilities prematurely will have unmet dependency needs and must make up for lack of nurturance at home by getting it elsewhere. Kind neighbors and relatives will fill these needs for many of the healthy siblings. Teachers may be looked to for such fulfillment by others. It is not too difficult for teachers to respond to younger children (kindergarten to third grade) in nurturant ways, but teachers of the upper grades are not so much in the habit of doing so. With the older child, there is a delicate balance between treating him with respect for his age and still treating him in a nurturant way.

Helping a healthy sibling starts with kindness and empathy, combined with a nonjudgmental attitude about the realities of the child's situation. Parents should not be judged. They are doing the best they can in a difficult situation and their healthy, normal children are loyal to them regardless of privations. The guiding principle in helping the healthy sibling is to do so without putting an undue extra burden on the already stressed family.

This does not mean that the family should be shielded from knowing that the healthy sibling is having problems. Once problems have been reported to the family, the teacher should work with the principal and other special staff to deal with those problems within the school to the greatest extent possible. Information gathering, classroom observation, and an interview with the child by the counselor would be an important first step, as the teacher must have some understanding of the child's situation and some clues about how to proceed. Information from a Child Study Evaluation may be needed if the sibling's problems appear to be complex.

PROBLEMS WITH SOCIALIZATION

Many chronically ill children must be protected from infection. Infection can exacerbate the disease to a critical stage or create serious complications. This is particularly true of congenital heart disease and sickle cell anemia. It is also an important consideration with asthma, leukemia, diabetes, kidney disease, and many other illnesses. Some parents, in their desperation to keep the ill child free from infection, will restrict their other children from any contact that might result in their becoming sick, which would in turn expose the ill child to infection. They will, in some cases, not allow social opportunities available to the healthy child and may even keep him home from school if there is an epidemic of any kind.

Brothers and sisters of a seriously ill child may be lacking in social skills because of restricted social contacts and also because of the protector and defender role they are often obligated to perform. If the healthy sibling must supervise and protect his brother or sister, he is not free to join in the activities of others. The role of protector and defender also creates barriers between himself and other children. Friends or potential friends may withdraw when a child physically or verbally protects his ill sibling from the teasing or rejecting remarks of others.

How the Teacher Can Help Healthy Siblings Develop Socially

The teacher should withhold criticism of siblings who are socially immature. Because of parental lack of attention to their needs, or because they have had restricted social experience, these children may be lacking the social skills of knowing how to gain admittance to a social grouping, how to show respect for others, how to accept losing a game, how to ask a peer for help, how to express negative feelings in an acceptable way, and so on. The teacher should instruct these children in how to socialize, using a nurturant approach.

Teachers, noting the sideline behavior, fighting, or social immaturity of a healthy sibling, will normally begin to think of ways to enlarge the child's social participation or to improve his social skills. This is a logical, natural, and understandable teacher reaction, but it must be undertaken advisedly. It is important to first find out the child's duties and obligations toward his family, as well as his restrictions. Greg was a boy who very much wanted to get involved with his peers, but he had too many family obligations.

> Greg was a ten-year-old boy who was in trouble for fighting and acting out at school. He had angry outbursts, talked back to teachers, and was in a fight almost daily at recess. The principal and teacher tried to arrange situations so that Greg would be included in games and social activities on the assumption that his

social exclusion was the basis of his negative behaviors (Greg was new to the school). However, Greg's behavior got worse instead of better! The kindly gestures exacerbated Greg's conflicts. He was an older sibling of a chronically ill brother. He yearned to be part of the peer group, but his family duties required him to come directly home from school every day. While at school, he was expected to look after and protect his younger brother. He did not feel free to get involved with his peers.

Greg's teacher could not automatically know the real cause of his behavioral difficulty. It took a psychological evaluation to discover it. In Greg's situation, the family reality was that he was needed to look after his brother. It was not advisable for the teacher to request that the family release him from this duty. It was believed that Greg could accept and carry out his family duties and adjust better in school if the teacher could offer him understanding and show him personal attention, provide for peer interaction within the classroom, and create opportunities for him to win recognition. The evaluation had revealed that he had a strong interest in history and was talented in drawing (although his academic skills were generally poor).

Subsequently, the teacher began to have short conversations with Greg whenever there was an opportunity. She talked with him about his brother, projecting to him a sense of pride for his helping role. She talked with him about his interest in history and learned what historical events interested him most. She found a book about those historical events that she thought he would like. She began to notice his drawings (he drew whenever he had a chance, but she had previously not been aware of this). She complimented him on his drawing skill. She created a small group project and placed him with several boys he seemed interested in getting to know. Later, she appointed him to direct the production of a mural in which the whole class would participate. In selecting him, she let the class know she did so on the basis of his drawing skill.

Greg's behavior improved in direct proportion to the teacher's recognition of his needs for (1) a personal relationship with her, (2) peer involvement that was nonthreatening and did not intensify his conflicts, and (3) recognition. Greg's teacher turned a negative school experience into a positive one by appreciating and respecting his unique family situation.

EXCESSIVE NEED FOR ATTENTION AND RECOGNITION

When a healthy sibling has high intelligence, she may strive to excel academically. The approval and recognition she receives for high grades and outstanding performance can, in some measure, substitute for the attention she has lacked at home. The healthy sibling can have unusual needs for attention when her parents have depleted themselves in caring and providing for the special needs of the ill child. If she has many talents, she may become a high achiever in other areas besides academics. Her high achievement enhances the family's esteem, as well as her own. It can serve the purpose of making up for what the ill child is not able to achieve.

With the child who has a need to display his knowledge, to act superior, or to otherwise make an effort to excel or "overachieve," the teacher should be tolerant and accepting. Some teachers believe they must correct or reproach a child for acting in a superior manner. However, caution and subtlety should be used in attempting to tone down such a child, recognizing his underlying need for approval and recognition. When toning down is necessary, it should be done with sensitivity and empathy.

Howard's teacher knew intuitively that his acting superior reflected his need for recognition. She helped him get it in a more appropriate way.

> Howard was a healthy sibling who was prone to use any opportunity to expound in an erudite way about information he obsessively collected. The information he offered in the midst of a class discussion often had only the most tangential relevance to the topic under discussion. The teacher ignored the behavior until it became annoying to her. She then took Howard aside and complimented him on his vast store of information but also told him that his remarks were often not pertinent, and that by making them when he did, he tended to disrupt the flow of the discussion. She invited Howard to give a presentation to the class on a topic of his choice, at a specified time, to be determined when he felt he was ready. She also said that he could give presentations to the class again later on, if the class had liked it and he had enjoyed doing it.

Howard's teacher showed sensitivity toward him by saying something positive before she criticized him. She created an opportunity for him to act important in an acceptable way. She gave him choices about choosing a topic and deciding whether or not he wanted to make a presentation to the class again in the future.

If a healthy sibling does not have the abilities or talents to be a top performer, she may attempt to satisfy her needs for recognition in other ways. Positive ways in which a child can gain recognition include volunteering for jobs available within the classroom or school, finding ways to be helpful to adults or other children, choosing unusual topics for reports, asking to do extra projects or reports, being appropriately funny or clever, showing creativity in art, music, or literature, and so on.

How to Handle Negative Behavior in the Classroom

The sibling who has developed negative attention-getting behaviors needs to be re-channeled into positive behavior. Negative behaviors comprise clowning in class, being rude, acting bored or noisy, being disruptive during group activities, coming to the teacher frequently even when help is not needed, showing anger if the teacher does not call on him to recite, getting into fights, finding fault with others, correcting the teacher.

When a healthy sibling behaves negatively, the class should be asked to refrain from reacting and reinforced for ignoring it. At the same time, the "clown" should be encouraged to use his fine capacity for humor in writing a funny story that he will be allowed to read to the class. A child who finds fault with others can be asked to write a report on everything he doesn't like about something he says he hates (a story, a certain sport, gym class, the school rules, and so on). This child needs to be given the opportunity to express negative feelings in a legitimate way, without directing his negativism personally toward others. For the child who comes to the teacher too often for help, assigning a work or peer tutor buddy may be a solution.

The nature of the unacceptable behavior should serve as a clue to the kind of task the teacher should create to turn the behavior into something more acceptable. Keeping in mind the child's basic need for attention, the personal acknowledgment of this need by the teacher will be correctly perceived by the student.

THE BENEFITS OF GROUP COUNSELING

Group counseling can be beneficial for siblings of chronically ill children. If the school system is sufficiently large, perhaps there are enough siblings within a school to warrant forming a group, especially as the ill brother or sister does not have to have the same disease. In smaller systems, one could consider bringing together the few siblings from each of several schools to form a group. However, these are new ideas, and a teacher will probably have to suggest such a possibility to her principal or the school counselor.

A report of a sibling group counseling program appeared in the magazine *Children Today* (November–December, 1981). Although the brothers and sisters of these children were considered "handicapped," some of them had conditions I have been considering to be chronic illness. The psychologist, Susan Pasternack Chinitz, started with the children by introducing a discussion about individual differences.[2] The children were asked to tell about their own qualities, likes and dislikes, strengths and weaknesses, and so on. Then they considered the qualities of their handicapped and/or ill brothers and sisters. Selections from books and articles written by or about siblings of handicapped children were read. The stories were the vehicles used to stimulate awareness and expression of feelings, both positive and negative. In response to the stories, the children shared their perceptions and experiences. Visiting the special classes of their handicapped siblings and participating in field trips with them was an additional aspect of the program, which took place during the summer. Information about the handicapped child's condition was offered at different points, as it became evident that the sibling had little understanding of his "special" brother or sister. The children were very receptive and interested in this kind of information.

It is possible that in certain schools and under appropriate circumstances, the method used by the psychologist in the counseling group could be used by a teacher, as the method is primarily an educational one. Children who are not siblings of an ill or handicapped brother or sister can also benefit from such lessons and develop more sensitivity toward both the ill child and his sibling.

WHEN THE ILL SIBLING ATTENDS A SPECIAL CLASS

When an ill brother or sister attends a special class, it is very important *not* to start thinking about a special class for the healthy sibling, even if his learning and behavior problems are quite glaring. The healthy child must be able to differentiate himself from his ill sibling. His problem in forging his own identity and in maintaining a sense of integrity and self-worth will be badly compromised if he is put in a special class. He will think that there is something wrong with *him,* as he knows there is something wrong with his sibling.

Ryan was a ten-year-old boy who was referred for a Child Study Evaluation because his teacher and the principal thought he needed to be in a special class.

Ryan was three years older than his brother, Eric, who was born with numerous congenital anomalies and a proneness to infectious illness. Ryan's needs from ages three to six were often neglected when the parents mobilized themselves for Eric's many hospitalizations, operations, and frequent illnesses. When Eric started school, he was immediately identified as a child in need of a special class. He had serious intellectual, learning, and social problems, as well as physical problems. However, the parents refused to allow him to be placed in a special class.

Eric, the boy who had never been quite right, was the object of teasing. Older brother Ryan was assigned to stick up for Eric and protect him. This created problems for Ryan because now he was excluded by his peers. The family had economic problems, and after many moves and marital struggles, the parents finally divorced.

Ryan had attended six schools by age ten. His mother finally and reluctantly accepted special class placement for Eric when he was seven. Finally, Ryan was free of having his brother in the same school. However, by this time Ryan had serious learning and behavioral difficulties, and the principal thought that he, too, belonged in a special class. The psychologist was adamantly opposed to placing Ryan in a special class. On a one-to-one basis with the psychologist, Ryan was an attractive, appealing, bright boy who showed himself to have artistic talent and a capacity for clever humor. However, he had a distorted view of himself. He thought his ill brother had all the personality and likable traits, while he, Ryan, was damaged and unattractive. Ryan already had a confused identity, having assimilated to himself his brother's characteristics, while assigning to his ill brother his own positive traits. The parents' efforts to believe that Eric was normal contributed to this process of identity reversal.

The psychologist believed that Ryan's emotional problems would become more complicated if he were placed in a special class. The family's esteem was also at stake. They were just beginning to come to terms with the reality of Eric's problems. They had anger toward the school about Eric's special class placement and believed the school was a rejecting, unhelpful place. Instead of thinking further about special class placement, a comprehensive plan was developed, based on the findings of the Child Study Evaluation, which was aimed at facilitating Ryan's adjustment in his regular fifth grade class.

By recognizing that the healthy sibling's behavior and learning problems are a reaction to the family tension created by the ill child, the school staff can direct their efforts toward understanding and support, rather than trying to rid themselves of his problem by pressing for special class placement.

Learning about the Ill Sibling's Special Class

When a healthy child has a sibling in a special class, he needs to be able to acknowledge the fact and to have some direct knowledge about the class. As with the children in the counseling group experiment cited, healthy siblings should be given some opportunity to visit and see firsthand how their brother's or sister's special class differs from their own.

Planning should precede the visit. Presumably, either the teacher, the school counselor, or the parent can take the lead in this. Naturally, the teacher of the special class must be involved. The form of the visit can vary, and this will depend on the teacher of the special class. Does she think it best for the sibling to come with his parent? If there are two or more siblings of the same special child, could they come as a group? Would it be more comfortable for the class if the siblings of two of the children in the class visited at the same time? It is possible that some special class teachers might establish a sibling visitation day when the healthy siblings of all the class members would come at once.

When the plan for sibling visitation is initiated by the special class teacher, coordination with the principals of the schools where each sibling is in attendance will be an important consideration. Parents of the special class children will also need to be involved at an early stage in the planning.

The Visit to the Special Class

The sibling's visit to the special class should be considered an educational experience for her. In some instances, the experience can also be shared with her own classmates. By reporting to her own class about what she has observed in the special class, a sibling will invite and encourage her classmates to accept exceptional children. She will give them a lesson on individual differences.

When a sibling visits the special class of his brother or sister, he should feel his own normalcy being reinforced. Perhaps he can begin to understand more about why his parents are so concerned with the special child. The privilege of such a visit will perhaps give him a unique kind of recognition by his friends. A child who proudly and publicly acknowledges that he has a special sibling will be more accepting of this fact and will be a model to his peers, showing that acceptance is a virtue.

There are some instances when a child should not be expected to report to the class about visiting his sibling's special class. In no case should the price of a visit be a report to the class. The sibling's visit is first and foremost to benefit the healthy and normal sibling. However, unless there is some reason not to do so, each sibling visitor should be asked if he wishes to report what he has observed and learned to his own class.

When a child feels shame and embarrassment because he has a brother or sister in a special class, he will most likely not want to give a report to his classmates. Tracy was such a girl.

> Eleven-year-old Tracy's adjustment problems were exacerbated by the fact that she denied that her younger brother was in a special class and pretended ignorance about why he went to a different school. She had gotten the idea that being in a special class was a shameful thing, and her embarrassment about her brother was great. Although her problems were complex, it was recommended that she be allowed to take a friend and visit her brother's class. For Tracy, filled with shame and embarrassment, it would have been too overwhelming to her to report to the class or to publicly acknowledge her brother as "special." However, by taking a friend with her, her "secret" about her brother would be shared with at least one other child, and she could begin to overcome her feelings of shame in a gradual manner.

THE SIBLING INFORMATION NETWORK*

There is an increasing awareness among professionals of the unmet needs of siblings of handicapped children, of which the chronically ill are a subgroup. An organization has been formed to respond to families and professionals regarding the needs of healthy and normal siblings. The organization is called "The Sibling Information Network." Membership dues are minimal and are used to defray the cost of publishing a newsletter four times a year. The newsletter publishes requests for information and experiences of parents, siblings, students, or professionals; descriptions of programs aimed at helping siblings and families; reviews of books and articles; announcements of

*For further information, write to the Sibling Information Network, Department of Educational Psychology, Box U. 64, University of Connecticut, Storrs, CT 06268.

conferences; in fact, anything of relevance that relates to the welfare of siblings of the handicapped.

WHEN AN ILL SIBLING DIES†

School children who experience the death of a sibling are at high risk for developing emotional and learning problems.[3] It is important for a teacher to understand how this particular child and his family are dealing with their grief. If they are mourning in a healthy manner, failing schoolwork or erratic behavior in the surviving sibling may be of short term. If mourning is inadequate or unhealthy, the chances are great that unresolved grief will result in long-term difficulties.

A parent who is emotionally bonded to a dying child may feel that part of himself is dying with the child. Parents commonly feel that it is not right to be alive after one's child has died; they feel that they should have found a way to sacrifice their own life for the child's. Surviving siblings are drawn into this kind of thinking and begin to believe that they too should not be alive.

Parents may deny their loss by displacing their affection for and expectations of the dead child onto their other children. If there is only one surviving sibling, the full load of parental love and expectations will descend upon him. If there are no siblings at the time of the ill child's death, a later-born child may be seen as a replacement and fall heir to parental displacement. A replacement child incorporates the ghost of his unknown dead sibling into the earliest stages of his personality development. A dual set of expectations—impossible to fulfill—and a dual identity will be his heritage.

The Burden of the Survivor

A surviving sibling, in addition to the burden of his parents' grief, has his own sense of loss to deal with. Whether or not the deceased child was a friendly companion or a rivalrous competitor, the surviving sibling's personality will have been strongly influenced by the pattern of the relationship. If the dead sibling has been a positive reinforcer of one's own value and esteem, the loss of the sibling will be deeply felt. Surviving siblings must reorganize their personalities following the

---

†Adapted from *The Sibling Bond* by Stephen P. Bank and Michael D. Kahn, © 1982 by Basic Books. Reprinted by permission of the publisher.

death of a brother or sister. This requires time and a great deal of emotional energy.

Surviving siblings, in their efforts to deal with the emotional whirlpool they are caught in, may display a variety of cognitive and behavioral difficulties as they try to cope. Some will seem unable to comprehend new material or will be unable to remember things they had previously learned. They may have distorted concepts of illness and death. A study by Albert C. Cain and others[4] showed that surviving siblings manifest a wide range of disturbances, including anger toward doctors, fear of hospitals, death phobias, and hysterical reactions on the anniversary of the sibling's death. If the sibling who died was older, the survivor may fear that he will die when he reaches that age. Parents may harbor similar fears and become overprotective of the surviving child in an effort to prevent another tragedy.

Parents frequently are so emotionally depleted following a child's death that they do not recognize the plight of the surviving sibling. Stephen P. Bank and Michael D. Kahn point out that parents commonly fail to assist their surviving children in healthy mourning.[5] The surviving sibling may feel like an orphan, deserted by his sibling and emotionally abandoned by his parents.

The Survivor as a Parental Distractor

The "orphan," moreover, may feel it is his responsibility to distract his parents from their feelings of sorrow and guilt. The child can do this by adopting the characteristics of the dead sibling, giving the parents the sense that the dead child still lives. The surviving child may, on the other hand, temporarily distract his parents from their grief by developing a "problem."

Brandon is a boy who developed a problem in learning math.

Brandon was seven when his fifteen-year-old brother died. The older brother had had a lot of trouble with math during his school years. Brandon began to have trouble in math. Despite five years of tutoring, his achievement level in math at age twelve was still second grade, just where it had been when his brother died. He periodically showed that he understood all math processes and that he could do seventh grade level math, but this only happened when his mother sat with him while he worked. In school, he continually did poorly in math, seeming never to remember what he had learned. He had few friends and did not go out for sports because he feared bodily harm. His mother was very protective of him and was afraid that he would be hurt if he played sports. Brandon had assimilated her fear. The family had never adequately mourned the brother's death. The mother continued to blame herself. The older siblings, now in their twenties, were having trouble leaving home. Everyone shared the family's self-blame and all were helping their mother keep from becoming too depressed. This was an educated and insightful family, and they were now ready to follow their psychologist's recommendation to work out their grief with a therapist.

The Need for Professional Help

Because of the extreme difficulty in achieving healthy mourning, families should be encouraged to use professional help when a child dies. The hospital social worker should be immediately available. Professional or volunteer bereavement support groups are also appropriate resources to use.[6] Incomplete grief will take its toll on most family members. However, the family may not be ready to acknowledge its need for help until months or years later. By acting when it did, even though it was five years after the death, Brandon's family was able to assure that its surviving children would have productive futures.

The parental stress of having a chronically ill child has been implicit throughout the discussion in this chapter. The specific things that parents must cope with and how they can be guided in their coping efforts are discussed in the next chapter.

NOTES

1. Gerald P. Koocher and John E. O'Malley, *The Damocles Syndrome: Psychosocial Consequences of Surviving Childhood Cancer* (New York: McGraw-Hill, 1981) p. 103.

2. Susan P. Chinitz, "A Sibling Group for Brothers and Sisters of Handicapped Children." *Children Today*, November–December, 1981, pp. 21–23.

3. Albert C. Cain, Irene Fast, and Mary E. Erickson, "Children's Disturbed Reactions to the Death of a Sibling," *American Journal of Orthopsychiatry*, 34 (4): 741–752, 1964, pp. 745–749.

4. Ibid. p. 745.

5. Stephen P. Bank and Michael D. Kahn, *The Sibling Bond* (New York: Basic Books, 1982) pp. 273–278.

6. Compassionate Friends is an international organization for parents who

have lost a child. There are more than 300 chapters in the United States. Parents can be put in touch with a bereavement group by calling their local mental health association or the Self-Help Center (see Chapter 9 under "Self-Help and Mutual-Aid Groups").

9

Helping Parents Cope with the Impact of Chronic Illness

Joan is knitting rapidly, while Herb stares silently out the window. They are waiting for the doctor, who is finally ready to report the results of Penny's tests. "Do you think it could possibly be leukemia as Aunt Mary suggested?" Herb turns around slowly, hunches his shoulders and says, "Good God, I hope not!"

Hearing the diagnosis is a devastating experience for parents. Learning that one's child has a serious chronic illness is always a shock. The material in this chapter tries to sensitize the teacher to the enormous stress that having a chronically ill child creates for a family. It also helps her to understand the coping-hoping process, and directs her in how to guide these parents.

INITIAL DISBELIEF

At first, parents have great difficulty believing the diagnosis. Mistakes in a diagnosis do occur, and in their upset emotional state parents can convince themselves that this is one of those times. Grandparents, other relatives, and friends also do not want to believe the diagnosis. They are also prone to suggest that a mistake has been made. Parents, although feeling dependent on the doctor and intellectually sensing he is right, often have a more difficult time accepting the diagnosis when those close to them insist it must be wrong. Almost all parents reveal that they have had to struggle hard with themselves to come to the point of believing and accepting the diagnosis. This process may take hours, days, or longer.

ANXIETY REACTIONS

The anxiety aroused by the diagnosis is intense. It can make a person feel as if he is going crazy or falling apart at the seams. One mechanism frequently used by parents in such a situation, to manage the intensity of their anxiety, is to repress the emotion stimulated by the news and to deal with the diagnosis as an intellectual event. Talking about the event in a detached way, they realize that they are feeling nothing. This inability to feel, to experience sadness at the time of the diagnosis and later during crises, worries them. Also, at particularly critical moments, upset at seeing their child suffer and feeling as if they perhaps can't keep going, parents may also become aware that very scary ideas are coming into their heads, such as "Maybe the child would be better off dead." They wonder how they can harbor such ideas and feelings if they truly love their child.

NEED FOR REASSURANCE

Parents need comforting and reassurance. They need to know that other people do not doubt their love for their child. They must be told that they *do* have the strength to cope and care for their child. They must be made to understand that they must not label themselves as horrible or awful for having negative thoughts. Fathers should be told that it is not shameful to cry or feel scared. Both parents should be told over and over again that their reactions are the same as those of other parents in the same situation.

Henry and Grace were a typical couple. Here is their story:

> Henry said he experienced every feeling from love to hate. He felt that the diagnosis of leukemia was synonymous with death. He was very scared; but when he saw his tiny son accepting the needles and painful treatments without kicking or screaming, he knew he could be brave, too. Every time a needle went into his son, it was as if a needle went into Henry's heart. It was so hard to see his son in pain and not be able to do anything to help him. Henry needed, and got, a lot of tender loving care, as well as reassurance, from the doctor and nurses. Grace was determined and optimistic throughout. She used the technique of keeping a daily journal to unburden herself and revitalize her hope.

In other couples, the husband will prove to be the rock and the wife will need reassurance from others. When neither mother nor father can take the strong role, considerably more outside help will be needed.

FEELINGS OF ISOLATION

When friends and relatives are very upset by the diagnosis, they may start to avoid contact with the family. They feel uneasy and don't know what to say, so they deal with their discomfort and uncertainty by staying away. Parents feel the distancing of their intimates acutely, but do not always understand the reasons for it. They may interpret staying away as rejection, which is unfortunate.

A strong sense of isolation is invariably experienced by parents when their child's chronic illness is life-threatening or carries with it a social stigma (for example, cancer or epilepsy). The isolation, the sense of being all alone, is often the result of feeling "This is happening to me and no one else." It is likely that the added dimension of rearing an ill or physically handicapped child sets them apart from their friends, whose children are bubbly and robust. They cannot share comparable child-rearing experiences.

FEELING DISPLACED

Parents of chronically ill children often feel helpless or displaced. It is their natural role to be in a position of authority, to be in charge of their child. When a child is seriously ill, this authority must be relinquished to others, such as doctors, nurses, physical therapists, and so on.

To a chronically ill child, the doctor is a hero. The child depends on his doctor for protection and looks to him for comfort and reassurance. These children identify with their doctor-hero as with a father or mother. Indeed, the doctor is a surrogate parent. A child may obey his doctor and disobey a parent, admire and show love to his doctor, while acting angry or hostile toward his parents. Child patients often aspire to become a doctor, or to marry one. They fantasize romances with their doctor and may become quite jealous of the attention the doctor gives other child patients.

The surrogate parent role that a doctor is placed in by his child patient serves an important purpose for the child but can be a source of hurt for the mother or father. The mother in particular feels rejected when her child wants his doctor rather than her for comfort and reassurance. Also, ill children frequently take their rage out on their parents at having to submit to medical procedures. This increases parental distress and exacerbates their feelings of displacement.

CHANGES IN THE HOME TO ACCOMMODATE THE CHILD'S ILLNESS

Parents must frequently rearrange their lives to accommodate an unplanned and unexpected diagnosis of serious illness in their child.

The cost of caring for children with the most severe chronic illnesses is beyond the capability of most families. The most serious illnesses require direct accessibility to a specialized care center, usually located in a university hospital complex. Unless a family already lives within commuting distance of such a center, it faces the necessity of moving, with all the adjustments involved in doing so. Sometimes it is important to move to a different climate or to change jobs in order to obtain needed medical insurance.

Less dramatic changes involve getting rid of household pets; setting up a mist tent in which the child can sleep (this may ruin paint and plaster); remodeling the house to accommodate a wheelchair-bound child; arranging space for testing urine, giving shots, or administering Factor Concentrate intravenously; maintaining a rigid schedule for meals; or organizing a time schedule for taking medication, testing urine, doing exercises, or taking warm baths. Roles of family members may need to be shifted and more flexibility developed to meet the needs of the ill child.

Changes in the family's routines, rules, and roles, as well as in the physical environment, must be organized by the parents. The children must be taught the new routines and made to understand why they are necessary. This will take time and require much patience. Explaining the reasons and necessity for changes will help the children accept what must be done.

STRESS ON THE MARITAL RELATIONSHIP

A serious illness or physical defect in their child tests a couple's relationship. Will the husband and wife pull together and meet the challenge? Will the illness prove to be too much of a strain on the couple's coping abilities? The high divorce rate attests to the difficulty couples have in making their marriages work under ordinary circumstances. When a marriage is already in trouble, with unresolved in-law conflicts or problems with rearing the children or career or economic issues, the added stress that a chronically ill child brings may be the straw that breaks the camel's back.

Another stress on the marriage is the parents' tendency to assign blame. Each may blame himself or the other parent. One parent may take the blame to protect the spouse from blaming herself—or put the blame onto the other to relieve herself of the anxiety it creates. However the particular blame system works, it is a normal but transitory phenomenon that must be resolved to keep the couple functional and supportive of each other.

The stresses that the marital relationship will suffer are not so different in kind from the marital difficulties of ordinary couples, but these in particular occur directly as a result of having a chronically ill child. The sexual relationship may deteriorate because one or both of the couple feels too burdened or overtired to be interested in sex; or they may start leaving bedroom doors open to be sure to hear a distress call from the ill child, which will also inhibit sexual activity.

Communication breakdowns develop easily because of the manner in which each parent deals with his emotions about the ill child. Parental needs for recreation and socialization may be ignored or denied because of the added care required by the ill child. Parents also often avoid socializing because of their sense of isolation. Financial strain because of the high costs of the illness may be another reason social and recreation needs are neglected. Financing the costs of care and of special equipment is a severe stress in and of itself. A multitude of worries can interfere with job performance, and concern about losing the job can compound the stress.

DOUBLE STRESS OF SINGLE PARENTS

Rearing children without a partner is difficult enough when all the children are healthy. When chronic illness is diagnosed in the child of a single parent, the family stress will be enormous. Several studies have suggested that families with a seriously ill child do not divorce with any greater frequency than the general population.[1] However, there are many single parents who have a chronically ill child, and the teacher must be aware of the double set of stresses.

Depending on the seriousness of the child's disorder, a single parent may need to consider who can be drafted as a surrogate partner. Is there a mother, father, sister, brother, aunt, uncle, cousin, or close friend who can assume the role? The financial burden, physical care, and frequent need to make difficult decisions can be overwhelming unless there is someone who can be counted on to share the responsibility.

Single parents in general have very little time to spare. They often have difficulty getting to school for conferences. It may be necessary for school staff members to reach out to the single parents of a chronically ill child by making home visits and helping them develop a dependable support system.

NEGATIVE EXPERIENCES IN THE HEALTH CARE SYSTEM

In addition to the ordinary sources of stress for parents, negative experiences in the health care system also occur. The total care of a chronically ill child generally involves several medical specialists and numerous other health care professionals. One study showed that a hospitalized child actually encountered forty-three different caregivers within a twenty-four-hour period. Within such a context, parents sometimes receive contradictory information, have things explained to them in ways they don't understand, get mixed messages about what they are allowed to do in the care of their hospitalized child, get pushed aside by an overly efficient nurse, have questions go unanswered, or overhear a resident complaining about their child's behavior.

COORDINATION OF MEDICAL CARE

Because of the number of medical personnel involved, coordination of care is very important but is often neglected. This leaves parents uncertain about whom to call when questions arise, or whom to consult when they receive what seems to be conflicting information or advice. The primary care physician (pediatrician or family practitioner) is the most readily available to the family, the one who has the most intimate knowledge of the family, and is the most closely connected to community resources. It would seem sensible for this doctor to be the medical coordinator,[2] yet many primary care doctors do not feel that the chronically ill child is *their* patient. That is, they feel that the child "belongs" to the specialist.

The role of coordinator is that of a manager and an educator. As manager, the medical coordinator must receive and send reports and maintain an ongoing evaluation of both the health status and the social and emotional development of the child.

As educator, the medical coordinator gives the child information about his illness in keeping with his capacity to understand. This must be revised and expanded as the child develops an increased ability to understand. As the child reaches an age where he is capable of assuming some responsibility for self care, he must be taught, in gradual steps, how to administer his own medical treatment. Children who understand their illness and participate in their own treatment procedures are the ones most likely to make a good adjustment to their illness.[3]

The educational role of the coordinating physician is initially focused on teaching parents. Parents usually need to have things explained to them many times because the emotional stress they are under disrupts their thinking and impairs their memory. Parents need to learn to give regular care, deal with minor emergencies on their own, and know when symptoms absolutely require a physician. Becoming competent in these ways keeps anxiety down to a minimum.

Unless one of the child's physicians has been designated medical coordinator, these important services may not be delivered to the parent and child. Parents should assume the responsibility for clarifying who is coordinating care. Teachers can encourage parents to be assertive and persistent with doctors, because it is in everyone's best interests to have a medical coordinator and to know who is serving in this role.

SUCCESSFUL COPING

The best copers are those who have had considerable experience during their growing-up years in successfully dealing with frustration or misfortune. For example, persons who have overcome a handicap, bounced back from rejection, faced disappointments and still take risks, or who have learned to have realistic expectations are among those who already possess significant coping skills.

Challenge, commitment, and control are basic components of successful coping. Facing an event as a challenge to be mastered; having a strong sense of commitment that allows a person to dedicate himself to others and persist with tasks in the face of difficulty; having a sense of his own competence and decision-making power and a capacity for some degree of control—these are all factors that contribute to successful coping.[4]

PROBLEMS THAT COME WITH ANXIETY

Even the most calm and stoic parent will experience immense anxiety many times during the course of the ill child's growing up. The normal anxieties of daily living are already there to deal with. Then, the anxieties created by the illness are added on.

Anxiety can cause all kinds of bodily discomfort and a wide range of physical symptoms. Keeping anxiety at a low level is important for maintaining health as well as personal comfort. As observable symptoms of anxiety also make others uncomfortable, a high-anxiety state can cause relationship difficulties.

A chain reaction is set in motion. As the mother's anxiety escalates, it is transmitted to family members, as well as to friends and others. The father starts to stay at work longer; a child starts to have tantrums; another acts up or fails in school; the mother acts irritable with the teacher who flares back negatively; and the chronically ill child's condition worsens.

EFFECTS OF REDUCING ANXIETY

In order to reverse the tense and overwhelming state of affairs, the anxiety level must be reduced. Deescalation of anxiety will allow for more effective functioning of all family members. With return of stability to the family, the children will act up less and grades will improve. Keeping the mother's anxiety at a reasonable level will facilitate everyone's coping, while health will be maintained, morale will hold up, and the ill child's medical problem will not become exacerbated for emotional reasons.

In order to keep anxiety at a reasonable level, the mother must become competent in dealing with medical crises; understand the illness well enough to make decisions and take appropriate action without undue reliance on either the doctor or the emergency room; know how to help her ill child with the many new adjustments and emotional upsets he will have; and be able to find quick solutions for the variety of dilemmas and unexpected turn of events that will arise. She accomplishes this by using the doctor as educator, reading books about rearing special children, and learning from other parents with similar problems by participating in a mutual-support group.

TECHNIQUES TO REDUCE ANXIETY

Despite all efforts to deal with anxiety at its source by competent action, there will still be many uncontrollable factors acting to increase anxiety from time to time. It can help to know what to do when the anxiety level has risen too high. In order to engage in self-management of anxiety, it is first necessary to become aware of the bodily messages that signal anxiety. Next, the current situation must be examined to determine the source of the anxiety. Finally, an active effort must be made to reduce the anxiety level.

Dr. Helen DeRosis has written a book, *Women and Anxiety* (Delacorte Press, NY, 1979), that describes in detail a method for self-management of anxiety. DeRosis believes that women generate a great deal of anxiety trying to meet the demands of a reality situation because what is required conflicts with their deeply ingrained "shoulds." Some of the things she suggests that will help reduce anxiety as well as minimize the physical discomfort and harm that anxiety can cause are:*

- keeping physically fit through regular habits of eating, sleeping, and exercising
- putting anxious energy to work by engaging in constructive activities, such as knitting, sewing, cooking, painting, building, and gardening
- discharging anxious energy through vigorous physical activity, such as running, dancing, swimming, tennis, and soccer
- reducing muscle tension through relaxation exercises, such as breathing exercises, biofeedback, and visual imagery
- engaging in transcendental meditation, or adhering to the practices of yoga, Zen Buddhism, or other similar belief systems.

THE PARENTS' ROLE IN HELPING CHILDREN COPE

When parents are able to keep anxiety at a reasonable level, the chronically ill child will also be better equipped to manage his own anxiety, for he is not immune to anxiety and needs continuing reassurance.

The parents' role in helping a child cope is easier if the mother can perceive her child as normal and different simultaneously. This is very hard for many parents to do. Instead, they view the child as totally different or consider him totally normal; that is, some parents treat their child as though he is *always* sick, even though he has many sustained periods of health. Other parents devote a great deal of energy toward convincing themselves and giving the child the idea that he is just like everyone else, that he is totally normal. Still other parents vacillate: At one moment, the child is viewed as 100 percent okay, at other times, as 100 percent sick, with no apparent correlation with his periods of sickness or health.[5]

A parent teaches a child to cope when she encourages him to meet the challenges of each new stage of development, allowing him extra time as needed and helping him face the hurts and disappointments that his particular handicap or restrictions bring about. He must be

*Excerpted from *Women and Anxiety: A Step-by-Step Program for Managing Anxiety and Depression* by Helen A. DeRosis, © 1979 by Helen A. DeRosis. Reprinted by permission of Delacorte Press.

taught what to tell other children about his illness or handicap, how to deal with the unkind words or actions of others, and how to make and maintain friendships. He must be helped to deal with his fears, anger, and pain, with the eventuality of hospitalizations and surgeries, and with how to keep feeling like a regular family member. He must be disciplined and given chores, be included in the sibship bond, and be taken on family vacations and other family outings. (Being included in the sibship bond means not being excluded from intimacy sharing with brothers and sisters.)

Books are a source of important information for parents. Audrey McCollum's book, *The Chronically Ill Child* (Yale University Press, New Haven, 1981), is a guidance manual for dealing with the special issues that arise at each developmental stage during a chronically ill child's growth.* Joan Fassler's book, *Helping Children Cope: Mastering Stress Through Books and Stories* (The Free Press, NY, 1978), guides parents to appropriate stories that can help a child deal with a variety of dilemmas. In addition to books that prepare a child for hospitalization and surgery, she discusses "Reassuring Stories to Help Counteract Fears of Abandonment," "Gentle Stories to Help a Child Relax at Bedtime," "Stories Portraying Some Inner Concerns and Anxieties Surrounding Bedtime," "Stories That Help a Child Deal with Separation" (separation fears arise upon entering school as well as when the child is hospitalized), and "Stories about Dreams and Dreaming."

Older children may benefit from learning to understand their dreams. For parents who are interested in this subject, Patricia Garfield's *Your Child's Dreams* (Ballantine Books, NY, 1984), and *Working with Dreams* (Delacorte Press, NY, 1979) by Montague Ullman and Nan Zimmerman are recommended. Dream work can help adults, and adults can teach children how to understand and use their dreams. When a person becomes adept at understanding the messages from the subconscious that dreams provide, a valuable tool for coping will have been discovered.

RESOURCES AND COUNSELING

If parents and chronically ill children are to cope satisfactorily, they must make effective use of available resources. The danger for a parent is to become too self-sacrificing or to deny or ignore his own needs, thus becoming a martyr. The hazards of overprotecting, in-

---

*This book is available from the Association for the Care of Children's Health, 3615 Wisconsin Ave. N.W., Washington, DC 20016. The association also publishes very inexpensive pamphlets that contain helpful ideas.

dulging, and becoming emotionally overinvolved with the ill child have been discussed in Chapter 5.

Some individuals are constricted. They shut out feelings of awareness, have a closed mind about new ideas, and often keep themselves at a distance from others. They have limited coping resources readily available when sudden and unexpected events occur over which they have no control. They will need help in discovering or rediscovering their hidden resources, such as intelligence, creativity, and sense of humor. A person's positive and hopeful attitudes, philosophy of life, and religious beliefs that help transcend misfortune are additional resources. The ability to be dependent or independent according to the requirements of the situation and the flexibility in using thought processes for problem solving are also important resources. Interest in and sensitivity to others, accurate social perception, and openness to friendly gestures made by others are personality traits that facilitate adjustment to illness.

Resources within the family have to do with flexibility in assigning and taking roles, modes of achieving anxiety reduction, and ways of offering support and comfort to each other. Creative planning of time, space, and finances; organization and mobilization of each individual's talents and abilities, including those of extended family members; and utilization of a variety of problem-solving strategies are among the ways a family makes effective use of resources.

Community resources extend from the families in the neighborhood to the friendship network and include all the established agencies of society: library, church, school, hospital, social agencies, government agencies, and so on. Of these, the library is the most often overlooked. However, it is an important resource as information is needed for understanding and for help in making decisions. The library can provide factual information to guide the intellect and stimulate thought, fiction in many forms to enrich fantasy and nourish the imagination, and poetry to involve the emotions. Literature and drama help one accept what must be accepted, and crying over someone else's tragedy can give relief to the unshed tears of one's own anguish.

Parents must keep searching for new resources if the ones already being used are not fully beneficial. Counseling is an avenue to developing or expanding an individual's or a family's resources. Parents who perceive counseling services as a way to develop resources or to learn to cope more competently are likely to be open to using them. On the other hand, if counseling is viewed by parents as meaning they have failed or that they are neurotic or crazy, they will resist any suggestions that they need this kind of help.

Counseling services come in many forms and answer different needs. Groups for ill children, siblings, or parents are one form. Counseling for the family unit is another. The sick child, a sibling, or parent may require individual help. A social worker may be needed to work out a plan of financial assistance, coordination of services, or transportation to and from medical settings.

A newer orientation of clinicians working in the sphere of chronic illness is to teach coping skills. A variety of coping skills have been defined, and these can be taught and learned.[6] Many family therapists include the teaching of coping skills within a more general framework of clinical intervention. Stress clinics also are beginning to emerge. In these, counseling is combined with teaching coping skills in a small group setting. It is not necessary that all the group members are experiencing the same kind of stress. Some professional practitioners are even offering stress training directly to children. The possibilities for teaching coping skills to children within a school setting are there, if the general public can be persuaded that this should be done.

Self-Help and Mutual-Aid Groups

Conventional forms of emotional help have not been available in sufficient magnitude or at a reasonable enough cost to serve the vast numbers who suffer psychological pain. Professional counselors have also lacked the experience and know-how to meet the needs of various special problem groups. Because of this, self-help and mutual-aid groups came into being. These are variously named: "Compassionate Friends," "Make Today Count," "Caring and Sharing," "Candlelighters," and so on.

Self-help groups are organized by ordinary people to help other people who have shared similar experiences. They all exist for the purpose of providing emotional support, guidance, and information to their members.

The most recent development in the self-help movement is the effort to establish regional clearinghouses that would ultimately become organized under the umbrella of a national clearinghouse. This would make it possible for virtually every community and all groups to have access to this kind of help. Individuals desiring help would be referred to an already existing group in their vicinity or be given direction in establishing a group.*

---

*The Self-Help Center, Leonard Borman, President, 1600 Dodge St., Evanston, IL 60201 Phone: (312) 328-0470, has established itself as a national clearinghouse and will offer assistance and information to anyone in the United States. Currently there are twenty-four such clearinghouses, and they are being developed in Canada as well.

The Professional Volunteer Connection

New forms of counseling and support services that reflect a merging of professional and self-help approaches are also emerging in many communities. These are particularly oriented toward helping the families with a chronically ill or handicapped child and those who have lost a child through death. They are family oriented, offering services to meet the needs of parents, siblings, and the ill or handicapped child himself. In some cases, these services are under the auspices of a local hospital. In other communities, an interested professional—doctor, nurse, social worker, or psychologist—has assumed the leadership in setting up special counseling programs and helper services for families having a chronically ill member. These programs operate on a shoestring. With minimal funds and maximal use of human manpower, a few paid professionals expand their helping capabilities by training and using a corps of dedicated volunteers. A major disadvantage for the professionals involved in this form of service is that they have to spend so much time and energy raising money.

An example of a professional-volunteer service organization is Project VIA in Modesto, California. It offers a variety of services. For families with a chronically ill child, there is an Individual Support Program and a Caring and Sharing Program. In the Individual Support Program, a volunteer, trained by the professional staff, is assigned to a parent requesting help. An attempt is made to match volunteer and client. For example, a volunteer who has reared a child with spina bifida may be assigned to a parent whose infant has the same condition. Whatever the need, the volunteer is available to respond to it. The parent requesting help may need someone to listen to her and respond to her feelings, to provide information about community agencies or specific sources of help, to help with transportation to the doctor, or to assist in filling out a complicated form.

The Caring and Sharing Program is comprised of groups that meet twice monthly with a professionally trained leader. There are separate groups for parents, adolescents, and young children. Members may have a child with any kind of chronic illness. This makes it possible for families having rare illnesses to belong to a group, whereas self-help groups are usually organized on the basis of members having the same illness, such as cancer, epilepsy, or diabetes.

Meetings generally have a prearranged general topic as a focus for group discussion. A member may report on a conference attended or on a book or article read, or a member or resource person from the community may serve as a speaker or discussion leader. Sharing of feelings is an important aspect of their personal exchanges. A quarterly newsletter and family outings offer the opportunity for contact and socialization between meetings. Families also offer support to each other between meetings.

Other services offered by VIA are a lending library of books, articles, and tapes; a bereavement support program; and the presentation of educational workshops for professionals or lay groups within the community.

There are services similar to VIA in other communities. What a particular program offers will vary. The imagination, determination, and commitment of staff and the amount of funds that can be raised will be determining factors in what is offered. Such programs are possible for any community. It takes leadership and hard work to get them established, but the beneficiaries will be the whole society.

HOPE

Hope is the fuel that keeps a parent going. Parents say that it is crucial to maintain hope even if one must grasp at a straw to do so. What does one hope for? That depends on the nature of the illness and the circumstances of the moment. In critical situations, a parent hopes that her child will live. At the other extreme, when a child has a mild disorder, a parent may hope for 100 percent normalcy. In this case, the hopes may be too high.

Dennis's mother hoped that an operation would make him as normal as other children.

> Dennis was a small boy with very mild cerebral palsy involving his legs. The doctor said that his walking could be improved through an operation. His mother was disappointed after the operation because Dennis was still quite clumsy. She had hoped for normal coordination.

If an illness or disorder has impaired the function of some body part, a parent hopes for an operation or therapy that will bring back the function. If the illness carries with it the possibility of serious complications, a parent hopes that these won't happen to her child. In the case of a degenerative condition, the hope is that degeneration will progress as slowly as possible. If it is expected that a child with a degenerative illness will be wheelchair-bound somewhere between ages eight and eleven, a parent hopes that her child can stay out of a wheelchair until age eleven. If an illness is life-limiting, a parent hopes that her child will live to the age of the oldest person on record who has had that disease.

Believing that a new medicine will be discovered, that a new surgical technique will be developed and of benefit, or that a way to halt the progression of a degenerative disorder will be found is an important way of maintaining hope. Religious or philosophical beliefs that encompass a beneficent fate will be useful. Praying is a way to ask for an optimistic turn of events.

Verbalizing hope gives it substance. If a mother is too shy to state hopeful wishes aloud, or if there is no one to listen, keeping a journal is a way to "verbalize" hope. Along with hopes and wishes, thoughts, feelings, and conflicts can also be recorded in a journal. This encourages awareness and reflection and can also facilitate problem solving, all of which are beneficial for coping and hoping. If possible, a teacher could suggest this technique to a receptive parent.

The more serious the illness and the more ominous the outlook, the harder one must work at maintaining hope. When faced with formidable possibilities and an unpredictable course of events, one can anticipate that the worst will happen, or hope for the best that is possible. Anticipatory grief is a way parents prepare themselves in advance for the expected death of a child. This process helps a parent relinquish, a little at a time, some of the emotional attachment to the critically ill child. Hoping continues during this process and will last until a child's last breath is drawn.

A narrowing of hope does occur, though. With a terminally ill child, a parent may hope that her child will smile just one more time, or that he will have at least one more "good" day, or that he will still be alive for the party the next day. When death is inevitable, a parent hopes that her child will be spared pain and will die peacefully.

PREPARING FOR A CHILD'S EXPECTED DEATH

Until recently, it was believed that children should be shielded from the knowledge that they are dying. However, it is now clear that children know when they are dying, even if the fact is denied by others. Anecdotal reports of children as young as two, two and one half, and three years of age verify that even these tiny human beings, who have no intellectual understanding of death, are aware of their own imminent death. Children reveal their knowledge of death symbolically, through both words and actions. The youngest children show it in their play. Older children project their knowledge in many additional ways, through drawings, poems, diary entries, sharing thoughts, and asking questions, as well as through play.[7]

Mutual Pretense as a Defense Mechanism

A difficulty for dying children is that even when they want to talk about death, they sense that parents and other adults are unable or unwilling to do so. There is a well-established ritual called *mutual pretense*, described by Myra Bluebond-Langner in her book *The Private Worlds of Dying Children*.[8] In this ritual, the child and the adults collaborate in pretending that the child will live, even when they all know that he is dying. When she studied dying children nearly a decade ago, Bluebond-Langner found that those parents and children who tried to deal with imminent death more openly were severely criticized and even ostracized by medical personnel and by other families. They paid a high price for their openness. Bluebond-Langner makes a good case for justifying the practice of mutual pretense. She believes that it is the way individuals strive to maintain the social order.

The Need to Acknowledge the Impending Death

In contrast to Bluebond-Langner's views is the growing belief that the parents and the child need to acknowledge the impending death to each other to help emotionally prepare for the ultimate parting. Many families may not be able to do this, and if they choose to practice mutual pretense, they should not be judged. It is the rare family who can discuss with their child his impending death without guidance and help. There are not yet many professionals who are prepared to help families in this regard, and even when parents want to communicate openly with their child, they do not know how to find someone to help them do this. Doctors frequently are not able to help because of their own emotional involvement with the dying child. A doctor may feel as if it is her own child who is dying.

Professionals who are experienced in working with dying children and their families are likely to be found in teaching hospitals of medical schools. Gerald P. Koocher, Ph.D., a psychologist at Boston Children's Hospital, and Aaron Smith, M.S.W., a social worker at Stanford University Hospital, are two outstanding professionals whom I have heard speak of their work. Dr. Koocher points out that a doctor should not be thrown off balance if his child patient asks if she is dying because if the child is *not* dying, the doctor can confidently reassure her. If she is dying, the child will not be surprised by anything she is told. She already knows the truth but wants to have it verified.[9]

It will be easier to talk about an approaching death more openly in families where the parents and the child have discussed death and dying at an earlier time, when no one was expected to die. They can build from these previous discussions. Wise parents are alert to their children's cues that they want to talk about death. As indicated, these cues will appear in symbolic form.

Elisabeth Kübler-Ross believes there is universal knowledge that death is a transition to another form of life.[10] She uses the metaphor of a cocoon as symbolizing a dead body, which opens to free a butterfly, to convey the idea to children that the spirit continues to live even if the body dies. This metaphor is easily grasped by children, and she has found that it can be very comforting for them to have this concept of death.[11]

The Child's Fears of Pain and Separation

Gerald Koocher says that the two major concerns of children are pain and separation. A child needs to be reassured that dying itself does not hurt and that everything possible will be done to keep him from having pain. A child also needs the promise that someone will be with him when he dies; in other words, he needs to know that he will not be alone. It can also reassure a child to be told that after death she will be with people she has known and cared about, including other children she has met in the hospital who have died, as well as deceased relatives.[12]

How the Teacher Can Help

If parents should ask a teacher how to deal with their child's impending death, I think it is important to remain nonjudgmental and not express personal biases. The decision about what to do must remain with the parents. Kübler-Ross's 1983 book, *On Children and Death* opens with a very clear and complete message for parents and can be recommended.

The teacher can also suggest how helpful it would be for the parents to have someone guide them who has had experience with this sensitive issue. Is there a priest, minister, or rabbi they know well? Have they been seeing a social worker or psychologist? Does the hospital have a person to help parents with this sad event? Do they know anyone who has experienced a child's death with whom they might speak? Is there a local chapter of Compassionate Friends, or another group of bereaved parents with some other name? The guiding principle is to listen sympathetically and ask appropriate questions that will point them in a helpful direction.

THE TEACHER'S ROLE WHEN PARENTS AREN'T COPING WELL

Parents who are isolated may well share their worries and burdens with their child's teacher. These are usually overwhelmed parents who are not coping well. The teacher must not get swept up by the parental anxiety, or assume the role of therapist. It is important not to further overwhelm such a parent by offering too many suggestions at once. First, find out to what extent the family has a support network. Is the family using hospital or community counseling services or participating in self-help groups? If not, refer them. Are there relatives nearby who can be asked to help? Do they look to neighbors for support or help? If parents do not have a support network, it is important to get one established. The teacher can alert the principal, counselor, or nurse to the need and together can generate ideas about how to get help for this family.

In order to maintain a professional perspective and without becoming overly involved with the parents' problems, it may help to think of the parents as being in need of "mothering." Comfort can be offered through tone of voice, physical closeness, and touching. The goal should be to project a sense of confidence that the parents will be able to cope. Helping the parents become aware of their strengths is important. Everyone has strengths, even those who appear weak, fragile, and helpless. Point out these strengths to the parents as they become manifest. Guide the parents through a "coping structure"; that is, show them how to set priorities, suggest ways to reorganize time and space, teach them techniques to manage anxiety, instruct them about community resources that are available, and encourage them to think of their own needs in addition to those of the dying child.

If an overwhelmed parent starts to cry or seems to be distraught, the teacher may help him regain his composure by giving him a paper and pencil and asking him to write. The teacher can say the following: "Everyone has hidden resources, and I'm sure you do too. Write down 'Hidden Resources; I must look for mine.' People cope, even when they think they can't. Write down 'I can cope.' Now, of all the things that must be done, think of the most important one. Write down 'Priorities' and the task just stated. The thing for you to do is get that one most important thing done."

It is to be hoped that this procedure will make the parent feel less helpless and more organized. It will at least keep the teacher from either dismissing the parent abruptly because she can't deal with the parent's being upset or feeling that she must solve the parent's problems.

The teacher's role is to support, instruct, and guide the parent in utilizing appropriate sources of help. The teacher should not provide solutions to specific problems, untangle emotional "messes" in the family, or judge the parental efforts. The teacher will be most effective with both her student and the parents if she can maintain this perspective.

NOTES

1. I. V. Kalnins, "Cross-Illness Comparison of Separation and Divorce among Parents Having a Child with a Life-Threatening Illness," *Children's Health Care*, Vol. 12, No. 2, Fall 1983, pp. 72–77.

2. Paul Steinhauer, David N. Mushin, and Quentin Rae-Grant, "Psychological Aspects of Chronic Illness," *Pediatric Clinics of North America*, 21:4, 825–840, November 1974, pp. 836–839.

3. Ake Mattson, "Long-term Physical Illness in Childhood: A Challenge to Psychosocial Adaptation," *Pediatrics*, 50:801–811, 1972, pp. 808–809.

4. Richard S. Lazarus, "Cognitive and Coping Processes in Emotion" in *Stress and Coping*, eds. Alan Monat and Richard S. Lazarus (New York: Columbia University Press, 1977), pp. 145–158.

5. Klaus K. Minde and others, "How They Grew Up: Forty-one Physically Handicapped Children and Their Families," *American Journal of Psychiatry*, 128:1554–1560, 1972, pp. 1558–1559.

6. Ethel Roskies and Richard S. Lazarus, "Coping Theory and the Teaching of Coping Skills" in *Behavioral Medicine: Changing Health Styles*, eds. Parke O. Davidson and Sheena M. Davidson (New York: Brunner/Mazel, 1980) pp. 58–64.

7. Elisabeth Kübler-Ross, *On Children and Death* (New York: Macmillan, 1983) pp. 126–144.

8. Myra Bluebond-Langner, *The Private Worlds of Dying Children* (Princeton, NJ: Princeton University Press, 1978) pp. 210–230.

9. Gerald P. Koocher, "A Child's Conception of Death," Kristen Hovda Memorial Lecture, Evanston Hospital, Evanston, IL, March 28, 1984.

10. Elisabeth Kübler-Ross, *On Children and Death,* p. 126.

11. Elisabeth Kübler-Ross, *Living with Death and Dying* (New York: Macmillan, 1981) p. 15.

12. Koocher, "A Child's Conception of Death."

10

Overcoming Barriers and Building Rapport Between Home and School

> Mrs. Boone is talking to herself as she stares at the note from Chris's teacher. "I can't believe Chris is acting up in school. He's an angel at home. I don't think Mrs. Green understands what he's been through. Naturally, he is going to feel bad when she's so unsympathetic. But I just know he wouldn't tear up somebody else's paper or purposely try to trip' another child. He knows what it feels like to be hurt. He would *never* try to hurt another child!"

Every parent wants her children to do well in school. When a bad report is sent home from school, there is the potential for tension and even friction to develop. Conflicts are prone to arise when questions of what to do about a child's problem must be answered. This chapter discusses the essence of barriers and how to overcome them, while considering how to build and maintain the rapport that is so important for harmonious home and school relations.

EMOTIONAL FACTORS

Parents of chronically ill children may well be more emotional than ordinary parents when they receive unfavorable reports from school. They may expect more of the school than other parents do. Problems between parents and the school arise if the school perceives the parent as expecting too much or if the parents believe the school is

141

not being reasonably responsive to their child's needs. Teachers can begin to feel that parents are not realistic and that they will not see that a child's problems go beyond what a teacher can do in a regular class-room. The parents may believe that they know best what their child needs and that the teacher doesn't respect their opinions. In these situations the teacher and the parents are likely to feel frustrated and misunderstood. This can cause barriers to develop.

THE PROBLEM OF BARRIERS

When parent or teacher feels negative toward, critical of, or angry with the other, it is very easy for a barrier to spring up. What is a barrier, and what must be done to remedy the situation?

Barriers block contact and impair meaningful communication be-tween people. They make it difficult or impossible to resolve dif-ferences, or for people to work together to solve their problems. Bar-riers occur in the psychological space between people. Fear, anger, distrust, criticism, negative judgments, and differences in values, be-liefs, or modes of communication are the stuff of which barriers are made.

Parental Barriers

Listen to some women in a mother's group describe their barriers. The leader has asked each mother to describe how she visualizes her own particular barrier. For those who had trouble getting started, the leader asked, "How high is it? How thick? What is it made of? How can it be moved?

For one mother, the barrier was perceived as higher than herself, thin but translucent, and flexible. She could not see through it or over it, but she could hear around it, and by bending it in from the ends she could see around it. For another mother, the barrier was low, but wide. It kept others at a distance. Seeing, hearing, and talking were possible, but not touching. Another mother had an accordionlike barrier. It could expand and contract.

As each of the mothers took her turn, the wide range of physical entities visualized as barriers became evident. A barrier translated into a unique nemesis for each mother. Depending on the "physical" as-pects of a particular barrier, the consequences were restriction of movement or impairment of one or more of the senses. Barriers re-stricted hearing, seeing, touching, talking, or moving. Barriers could be penetrated, but the difficulty and effort required to do so varied.

The constructor of a barrier usually expected the other to discover a way to remove or get around the barrier.

Here is a mother who feels that a barrier exists between herself and the teacher. She believes the teacher cannot "hear" her concerns, or act responsibly about her son's illness.

> Reggie Smith is severely asthmatic. His mother has been called to school time and again because he needed emergency medical attention. Mrs. Smith has made the principal and teacher well aware of the facts of the illness, but the early warning symptoms of an impending attack are ignored. Both the principal and the teacher are Christian Scientists. Mother believes that this is the reason the medical problem is ignored. She has become angry and frustrated, to the point that she can no longer talk to the teacher. She does not realize she could go to the school superintendent with the problem because her anger and the resultant barrier also block her from thinking of this possibility. The net effect of her barrier is to keep her away, keep her from talking, keep her from objective reasoning.

Teacher Barriers

Teachers can also be barrier constructors. This happens when a teacher becomes critical or judgmental about the mother's overinvolvement with her child; when parents won't accept the teacher's recommendations; when the teacher has not been given information about a child's illness; or when a parent makes unreasonable demands.

The latter reason explains why Timmy White's teacher became angry at his parents.

> Mrs. White demanded that teachers never mention to anyone that her son, Timmy, had cancer. Timmy missed a lot of school, received intensive treatment that caused him to lose his hair, and at one time was so ill he was not expected to live. The children were asking questions that the teacher felt she couldn't handle because she was not supposed to reveal Timmy's condition. She felt put on the spot and angry at Mrs. White, who had required secrecy about Timmy's illness. She felt justified in her anger, because it was generally acknowledged that the children were passing the word around among themselves that Timmy had cancer. No doubt, some had learned this from their parents. The teacher's anger blocked her from confronting Mrs. White directly about the issue. She also failed to discuss the matter with her principal, or with any of the special services staff.

OVERCOMING BARRIERS

No matter who is responsible for construction of a barrier, it takes a person on each side of it to help keep it in place. If a barrier is to be overcome, someone must initiate the process of removing it or moving around or across it. When barriers exist, people feel uncomfortable, hurt, or misunderstood. They are also likely to feel guilty because some degree of sensed responsibility is not being carried out.

Who should initiate the process of breaking through a barrier? There are no rules. The one who feels the most injured is *least* likely to attempt it. In practice, the teacher is perhaps the one who feels the greatest responsibility. She needs to restore contact, to get a problem solved. On the other hand, if a parent feels very uncomfortable and upset about the situation, she may be the one who initiates the process. It does not matter who takes the first step, but it will be helpful if both teacher and parent have had a chance to discuss the situation with an objective third party. The teacher has her colleagues and special staff members with whom to consult. Parents are inclined to use their friends or their physician as consultants, but they are not always objective or impartial individuals.

Barrier removal is never an easy process. Feelings have been hurt. People are defensive. Efforts to clear the air may be frustrated. Rapport, so essential for an effective teacher-parent relationship, is harder to establish once a barrier has arisen. However, rapport building must be the essential feature of barrier removal efforts. A series of conferences at regular intervals will be needed to build rapport. Problem solving will have to be delayed until mutual trust and respect between home and school have been developed.

Ongoing Conferencing

A plan for frequent parent-teacher conferences is both a solution for existing barriers and a way to keep them from coming into being in the first place. Parents who become upset at the first hint of a problem in their child should be considered as candidates for ongoing conferences. They are vulnerable; they view a problem with their child as a threat. They need understanding and time to assimilate the fact that their child has a problem with learning or adjustment. If rapport building begins before tensions develop or escalate, barriers can be prevented. It is far easier to prevent barriers than to remove them once they have arisen.

Parents may very much want such a series of conferences but may not be inclined to ask for them. Parents of ill or handicapped children may feel that they are a burden to others or that they are not deserving because they have had to ask for so much for their child. They become reluctant to ask for conferences, even when the need and desire for them is recognized.

The initial intent of ongoing conferences is to develop trust and mutual respect. In order to accomplish this goal, there must be a two-way dialogue and a sense of equality in the relationship. The teacher and the parent must communicate in such a clear way that their intended meanings are accurately received by each other.

In a rapport-building conference,[1] teacher and parent tell each other about themselves and their situations. They are people trying to get to know and appreciate each other. Each should share his own views about things that relate to children, such as education, discipline, child development, self-confidence, and so on. The child's school problems will not receive an intense focus at first. However, an exchange of information about the child is appropriate because he is the center of concern. The early discussion of the child includes a report by the teacher regarding how she sees the child in the school setting. The parent reveals what her child is like at home.

The Home/School Comparison

Is he the same child at home as he is at school? Does he seem to have a different personality at home than he does at school? The fact that children can be outgoing at home but shy at school, or misbehave at home and behave well at school is not outside a teacher's experience. However, teachers do not always realize that some children will act very dumb when they are actually bright, or appear not to know how to read, write, and spell when they are actually adept at these skills. It is not hard to understand why barriers develop when a child is seemingly a different person at home than he is at school.

There are different reasons that a child can function academically at home and not in school. For the chronically ill child, it may be that at home she feels secure and understood; she knows she will not be criticized if she makes a mistake, and she is not afraid to ask for help if she gets stuck. The same child may feel worried and nervous, shy and insecure at school. This can so inhibit her that she won't be able to recall, at the moment she is expected to, what a word says or a math sum is. Emotional blocking is another way to explain this phenomenon.

When the teacher is an information gatherer, she will not only find out whether the child shows the same behavior pattern at home as he does at school, but she will also learn about his medical problem and about his experiences with doctors and hospitals. She will find out about his relationships with family members and neighborhood children, and she will learn whether he has had problems in other settings.

The two-way dialogue offers the parent an opportunity to share the heartaches, frustrations, and burdens created by the child's medical problem.[2] As the teacher becomes more knowledgeable about past medical experiences and future treatments the child must undergo, she will be able to respond more empathetically to both the child and his parents. She will have the chance to see that some of the child's learning or adjustment problems may be an aspect of the illness or medications. She can also begin to see the connection between a child's anxiety or emotionality and his illness. In this way, parents can help the teacher discover how to best serve the child.

It is wise to involve both parents in the conferences if at all possible. With the father present, an overinvolved mother is less likely to be successful in manipulating the conference. Teachers should be guarded about giving advice. Parents who ask for advice invariably are the ones who find that what they are told doesn't work. The teacher unwittingly gives such a parent an opportunity to prove her wrong. In this way, the parent can disqualify the teacher as a professional and justify being resistant.

The Teacher's Need to Ask Questions

Instead of giving advice, the teacher should become expert at asking questions and at stating his own ideas as questions. For example, he can ask the parent, "What are your ideas for getting Billy to cooperate in school? Have you talked with Billy about his poor scores on spelling tests? What does he say? What do you think it means that Billy acts so sleepy in school?" Questions such as these convey that the parent must assume some degree of responsibility in finding a solution to Billy's problem. When the teacher asks, "Do you think it would work out in your family to have Billy do his math right after supper?" she is making a suggestion and setting an expectation in a format that is advice-giving without seeming to be.

Teachers should make it a rule not to expect parents to help a school problem child with academic work. Parents almost always create a conflict between themselves and their child, which exacerbates the school problem, when they try to tutor him. If parents suggest it themselves, they should be discouraged. If a child has no serious problem in school, that is a different matter. Parental help is sporadically sought by most children, and it is given naturally, without creating conflict.

DEALING WITH ANGRY PARENTS

Sometimes conferencing has *not* begun early, when a child's problems are of mild concern. Once the problem has become acute, and is reported to the parents by the teacher, the parents become angry. Conferences with angry parents will be most successful if the teacher does not become defensive. Angry parents may unload their upset feelings by attacking the teacher as unfair or incompetent. However, the confident teacher will realize that the attacking statements are just words reflecting how upset the parents are. The teacher must be able to hear something beyond the accusations, to begin to see why the parents are so upset. She will accomplish this only if she listens attentively, without becoming emotionally reactive, while the parents vent their anger.

In meeting with angry parents, the teacher should carefully create a setting in which rapport can develop once parental anger begins to dissolve. She should make sure there will be no physical barriers such as a desk between her and the parents, because she is aware that a psychological barrier already exists. She should secure several adult-size chairs, since there are mostly child-size chairs in the room so that she and the parents will be comfortable. The adult chairs convey, nonverbally, that the teacher respects the parents and considers them to be on an equal footing with her. She should remind herself that her postures and expressions can have an important impact. She should maintain eye contact with the parents and lean slightly forward as they are talking, to convey that she is interested and listening.

Before the parents arrive, the teacher should remind herself that she must not interrupt or try to talk too much while the parents are expressing their negative or accusing views. However, she should be particularly attentive to attacking statements, storing them in her memory for use later in the interview. For example, if a parent has asserted that Billy has never had trouble until he got in this class, at an appropriate moment the teacher can reflect this back as a mild challenge, "You say Billy has never had trouble *before?*" This puts the parents in the position of having to explain more about Billy's previous experiences with other teachers and usually shifts them from their angry stance. Another valuable way to help parents move beyond their anger is to ask for advice or information. "How do you think I can be helpful to Billy?" or "What does Billy's doctor think a good teacher would do?" are questions that convey respect for the parents' opinions, acknowledge the important position the doctor has with the parents, and express a willingness to be cooperative and helpful. With this attitude shown toward them, it will be very difficult for parents to remain angry.[3]

DOCTOR AS A GO-BETWEEN IN OVERCOMING BARRIERS

If a teacher has developed a collaborative relationship with an ill student's doctor, she can use him as a resource in preventing or overcoming barriers. There are important reasons for collaborating with the doctor, implicit throughout this book. Besides being a valuable source of support to the teacher in regard to medical issues, the doctor in the role of ally can become an intermediary between school and home when conflicts arise. The doctor is an ally of the family as well, so he can reflect the views of the teacher to the parent, and vice versa, serving as a negotiator or go-between. In this way, the dangers inherent in direct confrontation between the teacher and the angry parents can be avoided.

The Doctor/Teacher Barrier

Doctors have historically remained aloof in regard to involving themselves with school personnel. This is unfortunate and should be changed. Indeed, doctor collaboration with school staff is currently considered to be a vital aspect of good pediatric practice, particularly where chronically ill children are concerned.[4] However, pediatricians are sometimes at a loss to know how to make contact with teachers and counselors. Many do not know the full extent of the school's special services, and they usually do not know the details of regulations that govern special education practice. Some are prejudiced toward teachers: although they may not know their child patients' teachers, their own unfavorable experiences with teachers during childhood, together with negative reports from parents, color their attitudes. Negative stereotypes then justify keeping a distance from teachers.

If things are to change, I believe teachers will have to take the initiative in moving toward collaboration. Teachers will have to educate doctors about schools without threatening their dignity, and show them how to work with school staff in a mutually respectful manner. The negative stereotypes that doctors hold about schools will be dropped as successful collaboration takes place. Teachers will have to be tolerant if a doctor should act irritable or become abrupt or sarcastic during the initial stages of relating. They will have to be persistent in their efforts and show respect despite negativism from the doctor. Doctors are accustomed to acting superior and treating others as if they are inferior. Successful collaboration requires that equal status be accorded, each to the other, in the relationship. It will take doctors time to get comfortable with the idea of dealing with school staff on an equal footing. However, the teacher who expects to be treated respectfully as an equal and who conveys this by persistently asserting herself with the doctor is most likely to succeed in establishing a good working relationship.

As the initiative in developing a relationship with her student's doctor must usually be assumed by the teacher, the next section advises her on how to proceed.

HOW A TEACHER DEVELOPS A RELATIONSHIP WITH A STUDENT'S DOCTOR

In developing a relationship with a doctor, which will be mainly by phone contact, it is essential for the teacher and the doctor to have each other's phone numbers, addresses, and other identifying data. The doctor will also want to be sure he has parental permission for talking with the teacher.

First, Get Permission to Confer

The teacher's first step is to ask the parent for permission to contact the doctor. She should also ask the mother to fill out an index card giving permission, as well as the teacher's name and grade, the school's name, address, and phone number. The mother should give this to the doctor and tell him that the teacher will call soon. Then, the teacher should ask the mother for the name, address, and phone number of the doctor, which she records on an index card and keeps in a handy, readily available place.

Individual doctors have different habits about taking and returning calls. A particular doctor's usual procedure can be learned by calling his secretary or receptionist. The teacher should say that she has one of the doctor's patients in her class and anticipates that she may need to talk with the doctor from time to time. Does the doctor have a set procedure about taking and returning calls? If so, what is it? It could be that there is no set procedure, and the teacher will be told that she should just call when the need occurs to learn what the doctor is doing about calls that day. Depending on what is learned, the teacher will know to fit herself into the doctor's routine. One of the biggest difficulties in developing a relationship with a doctor is the frustration both he and the teacher experience when they try to reach each other by phone and one or the other is not able to take the call. The teacher should always be prepared to state a time and a phone number at which she can be reached and then be sure she is available at that time.

What Teachers Should Know about Doctors

There are several things that doctors feel teachers should know about them.[5] One is that the doctor would like to review the child's medical file or chart before discussing a child with the teacher. Whatever the pattern of receiving and returning calls, the doctor would like to be forewarned of an impending phone consultation with a teacher. The teacher should call the day before, or early in the morning of the day she hopes to speak with the doctor, to tell the secretary that she would like to discuss the student.

Another thing the teacher should be aware of is the doctor's reluctance to reveal too much. He must guard the family's confidentiality, and if he knows a lot about the family, he will not want to be chatty. He will feel a need for brevity in the conversation, so the teacher should think in terms of regular short talks with the doctor, over the period of the school year, rather than trying to get all her questions settled at once at the beginning of the year. In order to build rapport, the teacher must respect the doctor's limitations.

The teacher should know what constitutes a medical emergency, and if one occurs, state this at the outset of the call to the doctor. The doctor will always take an emergency call, even if it means interrupting his time with a patient. Determining what constitutes an emergency is perhaps the first issue that a teacher should discuss with the doctor.

Evaluate the Need for a Phone Consultation

As questions or problems with an ill child come up during the school year, the teacher should first evaluate the desirability or advisability of a phone consultation with the doctor before taking any action. She should then let the parent know that she would like to talk to the doctor about this or that. If there is any objection, this should be worked out between the teacher and the parent before calling the doctor. While thinking through a problem to be discussed with the doctor, the teacher should formulate a concise statement of her thoughts and one or more specific questions she wants answered or would like an opinion about. A doctor becomes impatient and frustrated if he cannot discern what it is that the teacher wants from him. He wants facts, and the main points of a situation being reported, not a lot of interpretation or speculation. The teacher who limits her remarks to a clear statement of a problem, followed by specific questions, will be well on her way toward building an effective relationship with a doctor.

Once the teacher has established a positive phone relationship with a child's doctor, the doctor will usually begin to feel good about having someone with whom to collaborate. When he knows that he can communicate easily and meaningfully with a teacher, he may even begin to take the initiative in calling the teacher for information. In overseeing a child patient's social and emotional development, the doctor needs information about what is going on at school. When the mother is a reliable informant and shares spontaneously how the child is doing in school, the doctor will not have to take the initiative in ferreting out facts. However, if the mother seems uninformed about how her child is functioning at school, paints a rosy picture the doctor wonders about, or makes many confusing remarks about school, the doctor will need a report from the teacher.

Helping the Doctor Understand School Reports

Physicians may be quite confused when reading the school's written reports of a Child Study Evaluation. A doctor may call a teacher to find out exactly what the report means. When doctors begin to ask teachers for clarification and for what the school can do for the child, the teacher is in a position to educate the doctor about the realities of the school and how special programs operate. She can also let him know what the roles of special staff members are and refer him to the appropriate person to discuss questions or issues that are not her responsibility. For example, the counselor would probably be more helpful to the doctor if he were concerned about a child's social and emotional development. If the doctor wanted to refer the family for psychotherapy, the counselor would be more familiar with local services available than would the teacher.

In referring the doctor to another staff member, it would be appropriate for the teacher to say that she could have the counselor call the doctor. If he is pleased with this and agrees, the teacher can pass on to the counselor what she has learned about communicating with this particular doctor. This should include telling the counselor what the doctor's habits are regarding receiving and returning calls.

WHEN BARRIER REMOVAL FAILS

When barrier removal fails, the child's problems remain, but with no solution in sight. Either the teacher or the parent may then seek to have someone else within or outside the school system intervene. Using the doctor, as just discussed, is one possibility. The ultimate conflict between home and school, in which the highest administrator supports a teacher and the parents are still resistant or uncooperative about accepting recommendations, will require intervention from outside the system. Sometimes it is decided that information from a Child Study Evaluation would help in settling the matter. The next two chapters provide information about the school's special services and guidelines about when and how they should be used.

NOTES

1. For more detailed directives, refer to Thomas M. Stephens and Joan Wolf, *Effective Skills in Parent/Teacher Conferencing.* The National Center, Educational Media and Materials for the Handicapped/Ohio State University, 1980.

2. For parents who want to become more effective in talking with teachers, there is a companion pamphlet to the above, Joan Wolf and Thomas M. Stephens, *Effective Skills in Parent/Teacher Conferencing, the Parents' Perspective.* The National Center, Educational Media and Materials for the Handicapped/Ohio State University, 1982. To purchase either pamphlet, write: NCEMMH, Ohio State University, 356 Arps, Columbus, OH, 43210.

3. Fred Wallbrown and Ferguson Meadows, Jr., "Working with Angry Parents," *The Directive Teacher,* Vol. 2, No. 2, Fall 1979, p. 10.

4. Gregg Wright and Nathalie Vanderpool, "Schools and the Pediatrician," *Pediatric Clinics of North America,* 28:3, 643–662, August 1981, p. 655.

5. Interview with William J. Morrow, M.D., pediatrician, Evanston, IL, October 1983.

11

HELPING PARENTS DISCOVER AND USE SPECIAL SERVICES

> Mrs. Kovac looks at her class list and the notes her principal has attached. Two children have speech problems, four receive learning disability help, Brian and Trudy see the counselor, and David, who has epilepsy, will be mainstreamed from his special education class. What does it mean for Mrs. Kovac when nine of her pupils are receiving special services?

This chapter provides information that should help a teacher deal with controversial issues related to special education services. Parents have gained significant rights of participation and disclosure with regard to special services for their child, which teachers and administrators must respect. Parental permission is necessary if a student is to receive help from a special staff member. Parents gladly agree to accept help that is educational in nature, but they are more reluctant to have their child be seen by the school counselor or psychologist.

Children with special needs were the "forgotten" children until twenty-five years ago. If they attended school, their unique needs received little, if any, consideration. Typically, they were excluded from school or kept home voluntarily to protect them from rejection, failure, or some other kind of hurt. In the intervening years, a number of events, and particularly the organized efforts of the parents of special children, led to the passage, in 1975, of the Education for All Handicapped Children Act (PL 94-142).

The purpose of this act is to provide that all handicapped children will have a free and appropriate education. In it, chronically ill children are referred to as those having a health impairment and are included under definitions of the Handicapped in legislation. The intent is to keep "special needs" children in the regular classroom to the fullest extent that is reasonable and feasible. This practice is commonly known as *mainstreaming*. However, the word *mainstreaming* has been omitted from PL 94-142 and replaced by the concept "least restrictive environment." The newer concept avoids the many misunderstandings that had adhered to the idea of mainstreaming.

MAINSTREAMING

Mainstreaming is the name given to the practice of keeping handicapped children in regular classes rather than placing them in special classes. It also incorporates the idea of integrating special class children into regular classes for a part of each day. It was never intended that *all* handicapped children could be maintained in regular classes.[1] The idea was to reduce the number of special classes by keeping the most mildly impaired children in the mainstream (the regular class). Many learning disabled and mildly retarded children can adjust and learn satisfactorily in regular classes. Some physically handicapped, blind, and deaf children also manage well and make progress while remaining in a regular class for most of the day. The majority of chronically ill children are enrolled in regular classes.

It is not an easy task to mainstream children with special needs. The regular class teacher cannot be expected to have full responsibility for special children.[2] A lot of help is needed. It is often necessary to have an aide in the classroom. The availability of a competent special staff is vital. Teachers must be given information about handicapping conditions, taught skills for individualizing instruction, and provided with the expertise for promoting the social integration of handicapped with nonhandicapped students. There are a variety of ways to expand teachers' skills and knowledge. These include in-service workshops, working closely with special services staff, and receiving quality supervision from administrative staff. Teachers must also have available appropriate materials for many levels of instruction within the classroom. A cooperative and supportive principal and the backing of parents and community are all important ingredients for making mainstreaming work.

During the early years of mainstreaming, many tensions were evident. Teachers were not given the help, training, and support required. Special children were returned to regular classes with no prior thought or planning about what was needed to facilitate their adjustment and acceptance. Conflicts arose over who was to have responsibility for the student, and for what. They were in the classroom but were still going to the resource teacher for help. Teachers were expected to grade the special student according to different criteria, and they were concerned about double standards. Mainstreamed students often forgot where they were supposed to be. Regular teachers did not have regularly scheduled conference time with the special education teacher who knew the child and his needs. Many of the requirements now known to be needed to make mainstreaming work were not anticipated. Except for the determination of the parents, the dedication of many educators, and the passing of the Education for All Handicapped Children Act, mainstreaming might quietly have vanished.

Teachers cannot deal successfully with the educational needs of regular and mildly handicapped children if they are pressured into having multiply handicapped children also. Teachers who resist taking the multiply handicapped deserve to be supported by their administrators and special staff. This does not mean that a child with extraordinary needs cannot be accommodated in a regular class; rather, it means that teachers who protest are legitimately asserting their own needs.

When children's impairments are such that it is not feasible for them to be fully mainstreamed, it is still possible for them to spend part of their day grouped with regular class children. These children are enrolled in a special class but may go to gym, music, or art classes with regular students. Severely handicapped students may be able to eat lunch or attend an assembly with regular students. There are also many special class children who can be scheduled into a regular class for one or more academic subjects. Sometimes such a child will join a class where children are somewhat younger in age. Age and size differences aren't as critical as many people think. Being on a social and academic par is what is important. This makes the special child comfortable and gives him a feeling that he can achieve success.

LEAST RESTRICTIVE ENVIRONMENT

The meaning of "least restrictive environment" is that a continuum of arrangements for educating the handicapped is necessary to provide for the variance from mild to severe in the nature and complexity of the handicap. This newer concept eliminates the propensity for people to believe that all handicapped children can and should be kept in regular classes.

Handicapped children who can remain in regular classes are

those whose extra needs can be provided for by brief and periodic involvement of special staff and by the backup help of paid aides or volunteers.

For the child who has special needs that require constant or continual help throughout each day, a special class in a regular school setting is probably indicated. Special classes for extremely handicapped children may be held in a building apart from a regular school. These children not only need continual assistance, but they are also children who have difficulty dealing with the total environment of a regular school. Other severely handicapped children may require residential placement in a hospital or live-in school. Most handicapped children attend a regular class, or a special class in a regular school building.

SPECIAL SERVICES STAFF

Whether handicapped children are enrolled in regular classes or in special classes, a special services staff is an essential requirement for helping to provide for their extra needs. These additional needs are educational, communicative, physical, medical, social, and emotional in nature. Special services staff members include special education teachers (sometimes called *resource teachers* or *educational specialists*), speech and language therapists, nurses, counselors, social workers, psychologists, and sometimes physical and occupational therapists. Doctors are often retained as consultants, but probably only the largest school systems have a doctor on staff.

The Educational Specialist

A teacher who has the expertise to adapt curriculum and to use unique instructional strategies with special children is called an *educational specialist,* and at least one is placed in each school. In very small school districts or sparsely populated areas, educational specialists who are resource teachers may serve more than one school, moving about as needed. The specialist is stationed in a resource room and serves the teachers and special students within that particular school building. It is possible that most if not all of the teachers in a building will have at least one mainstreamed special education student. These children receive individual or small-group help daily—or two to three times a week—in their weakest skills from the resource teacher. The regular class teacher should also expect to receive help from the resource teacher. The regular teacher should be provided with appropriate instructional materials for the special child and counseled regarding alternate teaching strategies and behavioral management techniques that may be needed. The teacher should expect to have consultation time with the resource teacher in order to accomplish necessary planning and exchange of ideas. When the teacher expects and receives these services from the educational specialist on the staff, he does not feel the burden of full responsibility for the special child. He feels supported and helped, and he learns new instructional skills in the process.

No regular class teacher should feel that he must know all there is to know about educating a special child. As indicated, he should expect that help and consultation will be made available to him. If a school district is too poor, too small, or too isolated to provide a special education teacher or consultant, a regular class teacher should request that his principal obtain consultation services for him. Special education consultants are usually available through the State Department of Public Instruction.[3] These consultants can also set up in-service training programs.

The Speech/Language Therapist

The speech and language therapist is another adjunct to the regular class teacher. A therapist may serve more than one school. The speech therapist aims to correct faulty articulation or poor habits of grammatical usage. She may work with a child to improve his vocabulary or to increase his use and understanding of complex language. She works with children who stutter, those who have unusual voice quality, and those who have very little speech, as well as those who have the more ordinary speech problems. A specialist in communication, she may also work with children who can talk but for some reason do not use speech very much for communicating. These children are sometimes referred to as *selectively mute*. Children for whom English is a second language are another group that the speech therapist works with. These children may have any of a number of language comprehension difficulties, although they speak English well, and *seem* to understand most of the time. The speech therapist works with children individually or in small groups, usually for one or several periods weekly. She should provide the teacher with feedback regarding a child's progress and tell her how to reinforce the things she is working on. The speech therapist may explain to the teacher how to adapt the language level she uses in giving instruction to be sure the language-impaired child understands.

The Nurse

The nurse is also a member of the special staff. A nurse frequently covers more than one school building. Although they have regular time assignments at each of their schools, they are always ready to respond to emergency calls from their other schools. Their duties usually encompass testing for vision and hearing, reviewing of health cards to be sure children have been immunized and have had the health examinations required by law, and overseeing the medical care of chronically ill children during the school day. If a child must take medicine while in school, the nurse is usually expected to supervise this. The nurse is also a skilled observer and should be consulted by the teacher when he has any question about a child's physical status. The nurse should be asked to offer an opinion (after sufficient observation) about whether a lethargic child is physically ill. She should be consulted if a child falls asleep in class, seems too pale, or falls down a lot. If the teacher has medical questions about a chronically ill child, he should review them with the nurse before deciding he needs to talk to the child's doctor. The nurse is there to serve the teacher as well as the child.

The School Counselor

The elementary school counselor has a background in social work or in counseling psychology. (The high school counselor serves a different role and has different training. The equivalent of an elementary school counselor at the high school level is a school social worker.) Counselors are prepared to help with social adjustment problems. They function in a variety of ways. They may observe a child in class and offer suggestions to the teacher about how to respond to misbehavior. They may see children individually or in groups to help them sort out mixed feelings, learn to deal with anger, learn to cope with the aggression of other children, and so on. Group situations offer opportunities to learn more effective socialization skills than they already possess. Some counselors—if the school system permits—conduct lessons in affective education within the classroom setting. Although the role of the counselor differs from school district to school district, the function of being a support service to teachers is invariant. One important way the counselor helps the teacher is to offer guidance to parents who are upset about their child's poor school adjustment, or who are in conflict with the teacher. The counselor also plays a coordinating role among the special staff and the teacher, involving parent and child in joint conferences when this seems wise to do. By showing concern for the feelings of each staff member, as well as of family members, the counselor facilitates a positive working relationship between home and school. The counselor is a member of the Child Study Evaluation team.

The School Psychologist

The school psychologist is the special services staff member whose role is typically to make a diagnostic assessment of individual needs. The psychologist serves as a consultant to all special staff members. The psychologist has broad training and can be of service in many ways if she has time and permission. Of all the special staff, the teacher probably has the least direct access to the psychologist. The psychologist may be based in the central office, traveling to individual schools primarily to perform a diagnostic evaluation or to consult with staff in a group setting. In a way, the psychologist's service to the teacher is indirect; she provides assessment data gathered directly from the child.

Depending on the degree of flexibility and creativity that a school administration allows its special staff, the possibilities for direct and indirect service to children is greater or less. A common complaint of professionals working as special staff in schools is that their roles are too limited, and the range of activities they may engage in is restricted. Rarely are nurses, counselors, or psychologists allowed to perform educative functions, although there are a variety of ways they can be useful in this regard. Special staff would have a greater sense of belonging and enjoy greater acceptance by teachers if they were encouraged to work along with teachers in classroom settings. Teachers sometimes feel that special staff people are so individual-child oriented that they do not give practical enough suggestions for working with children in a group setting. They would learn to do this if they could spend more time in the classroom.

Special services staff members tend to see themselves as catalysts. The unleashing of the energies and potentialities of parents, teachers, and child peers for the purpose of enhancing a special child's development is an important goal for each professional specialist. Even if it is their job to bring an individualized perspective to a child's problems, they are very eager to fit their recommendations into a teacher's realities. The more closely the special staff can work together with classroom teachers, the more effective they can be. Teachers who want to capitalize on the broad expertise of special staff members may wish to discuss possibilities with their administrators.

SPECIAL CLASS PLACEMENT

When children's special needs go beyond what can reasonably be met by the special services staff, consideration of special class placement will arise. Special class placement is necessary for some children with chronic disorders, and desirable for others. Unusual needs for physical care may be a basis for considering a special class, but wheelchair status alone is not a reason.

When a chronically ill child has social, emotional, learning, or behavioral problems in addition to his medical problem, placement in a special class may be indicated. Generally speaking, the more impediments to learning, adjustment, and self-care a child has, the more likely it is that suggestions about a special class will be made.

Special class placement should be considered when a child's behavior is so disruptive that his own learning is impaired and he is also seriously interfering with the teacher's ability to instruct the class.

When a child is having a lot of difficulties, a teacher will normally be in regular consultation with her principal and other school staff. All will work together to try to find solutions to the child's problems. When a Child Study Evaluation has already been done and all the special services of the school put to full use, the school will feel that it has exhausted its resources. It is at this point that special class placement will need to be given serious consideration. If it has been two years since the previous Child Study Evaluation was done, another should be done to establish the need for special class placement. Sometimes, special class placement will be the recommendation arising out of a first Child Study Evaluation. (The components of a Child Study Evaluation and all aspects of this procedure are discussed in the next chapter.)

The theory of mainstreaming has great appeal for the parents of special children, but the reality for a special child who remains in a regular class is often discrepant with theoretical expectations. Sometimes a child who has been placed back in the regular class will ask to be returned to the special class. He is indicating that he felt more comfortable while there.

The special class can be a haven for children who are chosen to be there. The pace and pressures are different, suited to each child's needs. There are fewer classmates, and each one has some kind of problem; the child is not alone in that. Competition is replaced by an emphasis on individual development. The teacher has an unusual interest in and a desire to reach out to children with special needs. Children who do not speak clearly, who do not express themselves easily, who cannot hear or see as well as others, who take much longer than usual to do work, who are clumsy or awkward in walking or writing, who tire easily, who get upset by criticism, who do not understand directions well, who cannot remember what they are supposed to do or where materials are kept, who do not handle their temper well, or who look, act, or think differently than others usually feel a sense of relief once they have had a chance to get used to the unique environment of a special class.

There is a lot of emotionality about the special class among groups of parents and teachers in some communities. These parents and teachers believe that special class placement marks a child and limits his opportunities for friends, normal activities, and education in the future. On the other hand, children who have been in special classes often prefer it to being in regular classes. There they get the appropriate attention to their special needs that makes them feel protected, cared about, and worthy. They do not always have to be striving to live up to "normal" expectations. They can be themselves and have the time needed to grow up at a comfortable pace. They do not *have* to feel hurried and pushed.

There are many stories that circulate about the lack of behavioral control of children in special classes, about the poor education children receive there, and about how difficult it is to get a child removed from a special class, even when parents have good evidence that he is not progressing and developing properly from being there. Of course, all of these things do happen; but how frequently? People tend to overgeneralize. School systems vary in quality. It is possible that where regular education is of poor quality, special classes will not be good places for children either.

The philosophy of normalization that permeates our current educational thinking dictates that special class placement should be considered only after all of the usual resources of the school have been exhausted. As with all difficult decisions, there are pros and cons about special class placement for any particular child. However, if a full staff of professionals is in agreement that special class placement is the best plan for a child, how can it be so harmful? In the communities where parents and teachers view special classes positively, people take pride in the fact that special classes are available. They believe that children benefit from the opportunities provided in special classes. Parents and teachers of all children, regular and special, work together to foster acceptance of the special class child and to assure that he can participate in normal activities to the extent he is able. The child remains in the special class until he can be successfully mainstreamed for one class period at a time. He is not rushed into mainstreaming. Parents who have been conditioned to be negative and apprehensive about a special class will need a lot of support and encouragement if such a placement is recommended. Teachers who know what goes on in special classes and have respect for the education children receive there are in a position to offer support to parents. Most schools have one or more special classes within any one building. Teachers of regular classes should talk with the special class teachers, listen to their views, and be aware of the kinds of children enrolled there and the kinds of learning they do.

Special education costs money—possibly two to five times as much as regular classes cost. For this reason, only the children who truly need this kind of expenditure can qualify for a special class.

WHO DECIDES ELEGIBILITY FOR SPECIAL CLASS PLACEMENT?

Special class placement is regulated by state and federal laws. These laws have set up a procedure that assures that very careful thought and care will be given in determining whether a child is eligible for a special class. Neither a teacher nor a school principal can decide to put a child in a special class—nor can any other administrator. The decision about special class placement is a joint decision in which the parents participate.

The principal, after a teacher has consulted with her about a child's problems, is usually the person who sets the wheels in motion that ultimately result in a determination about eligibility. A team of specialists then gather and evaluate a great deal of data (see Chapter 12). On the basis of the team's analysis of the data, a child will either be declared eligible or ineligible for a special class. If the child is eligible, special class placement will be recommended to the parents. The parents have the final decision regarding accepting the placement. If they reject the placement and the school believes that it cannot provide the child with an adequate and appropriate education in a regular class, the school may take the parents to a hearing.[4] School personnel and parents have the right to present evidence at such a hearing. The outcome is decided by impartial hearing officers who have no personal interest in the situation. If the hearing officers declare that the child must be in a special class, the parents will be required to abide by the school's recommendation for special class placement, even though they continue to object. If the hearing officer decides in the parents' favor, the school will be obliged to allow the child to remain in a regular class.

Parents also have a right to initiate a due process hearing. When they believe that their child is not receiving the services stipulated by law, or they have grievances about their child's educational placement, they may bring the school to a hearing.[5]

When parents are presented with the findings and recommendations of a Child Study Evaluation, they are invited to express their reactions. Do they agree with the conclusions reached, and do they think the observations of the staff and the test data give an accurate picture of their child? If special class placement is recommended, it is expected that parents will have questions as well as worries and concerns about such a placement for their child. Each of their concerns will be taken seriously and views of the staff given in response. They will be told that they do not have to accept the placement until they have had a chance to visit the class being recommended. A visit to the class and meeting the teacher allays fears more readily and more definitely than hours of talk. When parents see the children enrolled in the special class, observe the educational program they receive, and see the quality of the teacher's instruction, they are usually ready to agree that the class is appropriate for their child. After being given a firsthand chance to judge and evaluate the special class, parents feel more comfortable in making their decision about the recommendation.

If parents have not had a chance to visit the special class being recommended before the opening of the school year, they may be asked to keep their child out of school for a few days, pending the final decision about placement. It is psychologically unwise to pressure parents into accepting such a placement without giving them a chance to visit the class, but when parents do not question the placement and decline the invitation to visit the class, they should not be forced to do so.

It is important for teachers not to be critical of a parent who starts her child late, having rejected special class placement after the beginning of the year visit. The teacher must not let her feelings about the parents' decision interfere with acceptance of the child. Parents are exercising their legal right in rejecting placement.

Whether children are enrolled in a special class or mainstreamed, the real aim is for them to be understood, accepted, and included in social and recreational activities by normal children. It is also important that they receive an education that is in keeping with their needs and, at the same time, makes their minds stretch and grow. Opponents of special classes may think that children attending them are not sufficiently challenged. This may have been a valid criticism in the early days of special education because teachers were often not properly trained, nor were appropriate facilities and materials provided. This is no longer the case. Before anyone tried to educate the most seriously handicapped, little was known about how much they could learn. It is now known that they can learn more than anyone suspected. I believe that for appropriately placed children a good education is now possible in special classes.

GUIDING PARENTS TO USE SPECIAL SERVICES

Parental permission is necessary for a child to be taken out of class for any special service (other than screening tests). At the beginning of school in the fall, the speech therapist screens children from all classes who appear to have a speech problem. She then informs the parent of the child's need for help. Parents rarely refuse this kind of help because they are quite anxious to have their child speak correctly. Tutoring help from a learning disability specialist or a resource room teacher is given only if a child qualifies for it on the basis of a Child Study Evaluation. Parental agreement must be obtained to do the evaluation. Some parents refuse and others are quite reluctant about agreeing to it. However, few parents turn down tutoring help when it is offered. Counseling usually requires only the teacher's request, the counselor's agreement, and the parents' permission. However, some parents have reservations about counseling, and it is not uncommon for them to refuse this kind of help for their child. Teachers who persist in trying to obtain parental permission are often ultimately successful. In most instances, the teacher knows the parents best and can play a significant role in obtaining permission from reluctant parents. Here I will discuss the steps to take with parents who do not at first grant permission for their child to receive counseling. (The teacher's role in obtaining parental permission for a Child Study Evaluation is discussed in the next chapter.)

PERMISSION FOR COUNSELING

No matter what reason they give, parental refusal of counseling usually has to do with personal biases, distrust, and fear that family problems will be disclosed. Family esteem is also a factor. If a child has a problem needing a counselor's attention, it can mean (to the parents) that there is something wrong with the family—the parents have not done a good job of parenting. Parents may also be concerned that their child will lose his friends. These parents seem to think that counseling marks the child as psychologically "not all right" and that others will shun him. Although mental health professionals have learned from wide experience that these are the bases of parental refusal for school counseling, parents may not want to say so, and they may offer many more ordinary, flimsy excuses. This is a trap for teachers; if they take these excuses at face value, they will be inclined to offer explanations and reassurances that can put parents on the defense.

Few parents who are adamantly against counseling will change their minds, and the teacher should not pressure them or try to get them to agree. However, it does no harm to suggest that they think about talking with the counselor about it if they have not already done this. It will take something as dramatic as a family crisis or the threat of special class placement to get these parents to agree to counseling. If parents refuse but are less sure about the position they have taken, the teacher is advised to be persistent. They are the ones who may reconsider.

When the teacher perceives any uncertainty in the parent, for example, if the mother says, "It's all right with me, but my husband objects," she should urge the mother to talk with the counselor. Often parental agreement for counseling is given after the mother or both parents together have formed a relationship with the counselor. They may need to share certain delicate family matters with the counselor (that they don't want the teacher to know) before they feel trusting enough to have the counselor work with their child. They may need to learn the counselor's views about children and families and the way she works with children before they can feel comfortable about having their child engage in counseling. They may have had bad experiences with counselors in other settings and this may have created a degree of distrust that might otherwise not have existed. When they learn to know and respect this counselor, they can perhaps begin to trust again.

The teacher does not try to convince reluctant parents that their child needs counseling, but she does persist in recommending it and continues to state how she believes it could help. She should always be on the lookout for the ambivalent statement, for the point at which the parent acts uncertain. This is when she should try to persuade the parents to at least talk it over with the counselor.

Many teachers have had psychology courses and pride themselves on their knowledge of the dynamics of human behavior. They may be tempted to deal with the parents' ambivalence themselves rather than send them on to the counselor. These teachers must remember that no matter how skilled they are in psychological matters, the parents may not want to share intimate family matters with them. The teacher is most effective and also saves herself from potential negative parental reactions when she respects the specific expertise and role function of her fellow staff members. Referring a parent to the counselor rather than trying to deal with all issues independently is the mark of a mature teacher.

Children who are referred for counseling services are those who have obvious behavioral or emotional difficulties. When a child has learning problems and the teacher has not been able to pinpoint the cause or find a solution, a Child Study Evaluation is indicated. The next chapter defines this procedure in detail.

NOTES

1. Ann P. Turnbull and Jane B. Schulz, *Mainstreaming Handicapped Students: A Guide for the Classroom Teacher* (Boston: Allyn and Bacon, 1979) p. 53.

2. Turnbull and Schulz, *Mainstreaming,* p. 52.

3. Turnbull and Schulz, *Mainstreaming,* p. 68.

4. Public Law 94-142—Education for All Handicapped Children Act (Federal Register, 1977; became effective October 1977).

5. Ibid.

12

The Child Study Evaluation: How to Obtain Parental Consent

> Mrs. Platte is concerned about Barry. He never smiles and always seems lethargic. He gets little done unless she sits with him while he works, and all his skills are far below the level needed for fifth grade. Of course, he has cancer, but he hasn't been sick for two years. Yet before that he had operations and radiation to his head and was expected to die on more than one occasion. What does Barry need? Counseling, grade retention, tutoring, special class, or what?

Mrs. Platte consulted her principal, and together they decided Barry should have a Child Study Evaluation. The goal of the evaluation would be to get an assessment of Barry's skills and abilities, as well as of his unique needs. It would also show whether he needed a special class. Although the Child Study Evaluation is a necessary first step if special class placement is to be considered, the information from the study is most frequently used to help a child learn while he remains in the regular class. This chapter explains the components of the evaluation and what can be learned from the parts as well as the whole. The teacher plays a significant role in obtaining parental permission for the evaluation and in instructing parents to prepare their child to be tested.

Child Study Evaluation has become commonplace as an adjunct to wise school programming for children who have special needs. The timing of the evaluation is based on the need for information. A teacher might reasonably feel overwhelmed by the special needs of a child entering her class after a long illness during which the child was too sick to do schoolwork. If the illness or surgery involved the brain, she has further reason to be apprehensive. Frequent absences of shorter duration, characteristic of the severe asthmatic and diabetic child, usually cause the child to fall behind in his work. Is it only missed schooling that is causing a lag in achievement, or are there additional factors operating that should receive attention? The frequently absent child who is bright and motivated will usually be able to make up the missed work and move ahead at a regular pace with the class. But the less adept student or the one who feels he should not have to make up missed work will have trouble keeping up.

COMPONENTS OF THE CHILD STUDY EVALUATION

The teacher will feel supported and less anxious about receiving the long absent or frequently absent child into her class if she has some information about his abilities, his levels of achievement in basic skills, his style of learning, his motivation, and his ability to concentrate and become involved in learning tasks.

The Child Study Evaluation is the first step to take in assessing individual needs and is one way of answering the questions posed in Chapter 6, when a child is having problems with learning. The components of this comprehensive gathering of information about a child follow.

Vision and Hearing Testing

The school nurse administers vision and hearing tests to all students at regular intervals. This screening process identifies those students whose sight and hearing are adequate and those who have problems. Recent reports of examinations done privately or by a public health agency are other sources of information.

Typically, when children are shown to have problems with vision or hearing, the school nurse will monitor them to be sure these problems are receiving appropriate care and regular evaluation by a physician. As indicated in Chapter 6, a child's learning problem (particularly not paying attention) may be wholly or partially explained on the basis of a vision or hearing problem. The teacher should check with the school nurse to determine whether the child is hearing and seeing adequately. Obviously, the teacher does not have to initiate a Child Study Evaluation in order to get an up-to-date screening of vision and hearing, but testing of these sense organs is always a component of the Child Study Evaluation. Hearing and vision tests determine whether a child has normal function of his ears and eyes. They do not determine whether he has auditory or visual perceptual problems, nor do they determine if the child has poor habits of listening and looking. Problems with the manner in which a child uses his ears and eyes for learning are detected through the educational and perceptual tests that are administered by either an educational specialist or a school psychologist.

Health History

Typically, a form is filled out by the parent or by the counselor or school nurse interviewing the parents. The questions on the form ask for details of birth history, illnesses, accidents, hospitalizations, medications, surgeries, allergies, handicaps, and so on. Health problems in other family members are also of important concern.

This information is important for understanding a child's physical problems as well as the psychological impact that illness, either his own or that of a close family member, has had on him. If there has been a difficult birth or serious illness in the first year of life, it could have resulted in subtle changes in the brain that impair learning. Perhaps frequent ear infections or chronic allergic reactions have been accompanied by recurrent periods when the child did not hear well. This could affect the development of his habits of listening and his learning to discriminate auditory stimuli as well as the development of his speech, language, and vocabulary. Perhaps there have been visual problems in the past, which are now corrected. These could have delayed the development of certain visual skills needed for learning; for example, looking carefully at fine detail, and visual scanning. Any health impairment that could have delayed development or any traumatic medical experience that could have caused emotional problems will need to be evaluated carefully.

Child Development/Family History

An interview with the parents is held by the school counselor (or perhaps the school psychologist) to elicit information about a child's development and his experiences of living within the family.

Taking the health history is often combined with this interview. The counselor will invite both parents to come in. When both parents are present, a more complete picture of the child's life xperiences can be obtained. Both parents are expected at the report conference when test findings are explained, and it provides continuity for them when they both participate from the beginning. In addition to such questions as when the child learned to walk, talk, use the toilet, and dress himself, the counselor will be looking for clues about the family's value system, modes of discipline, attitudes about child-rearing issues that can be related to school functioning, how the parents view the child's personality, temperament, and so on. Significant family history information includes an overview of the parents' growing-up experiences in their families, a description of present contact with the grandparent generation, and whether or not parents or close family members had reading or other learning problems during their school years. Patterns of intrafamily relating and ways of dealing with conflict tend to be repeated from generation to generation. Knowing what these patterns were in the parents' families can help in perceiving the repetition of the patterns in the current generation of which the child is a part.

Report from the Teacher

The teacher writes a statement regarding the nature of the child's problems, what she has done to help the child, and at what academic level she estimates the child to be achieving. If the child is having behavioral problems, she also describes these and tells what she has done to help and how the child has reacted.

The teacher is the closest daily observer of the child while he is in school, and she knows a great deal about him. However, like a parent, the teacher sometimes loses her objectivity about the child because of her involvement with him. The teacher may not be aware of biases she has about the child's words and actions (for example, she may interpret what he says and does from a stance of assumptions and prejudgments). In giving her report, the teacher is encouraged to express her opinions and attitudes toward the child. This will help the staff determine whether her words and actions are part of the problem and in need of being modified. It is assumed by the professional staff that teachers, like parents, always want to do what is best for a child. However, our humanness sometimes impairs our ability to do so. The goal of the evaluation—to discover the source of a child's problem and what to do about it—must be kept in the foreground of the teacher's thinking. Otherwise, she might become defensive if one of the special staff or a parent suggests a way of dealing with the child that is different from her usual way.

Observation of the Child in Class

One or more of the evaluation team members (counselor, psychologist, educational specialist) observes the child during a regular class period.

The observer will watch what the child is doing while the teacher is delivering instruction: Is he attending? Does he respond appropriately when called on? How does he get settled down to work? Does he seem to understand what is going on? How does he react when he is corrected? How do other children react or relate to him; that is, is he respected or ridiculed?

The observer stays long enough to see the child function in a variety of situations. Perhaps he will read orally, recite, or do a math paper or other seat work while the observer is present. An effort is usually made to do the observation without making the child aware that he is the one being observed. By having an independent observation of the child's behavior in class, the teacher's report of the child's usual behavior can be validated or questioned.

School History

The parent is asked to list the schools her child has attended; the grades repeated; the problems with learning that have been previously suggested; whether the child has received any tutorial help, counseling; and so on. This gives the evaluation team a chance to consider the kinds of stresses a child has had that are directly related to the school experience. A child who has moved a lot has had to adjust to many different schools as well as to a variety of modes of class grouping and patterns of instruction. He could have many gaps in his skills either because of missed sequences of instruction or because difficulties in adjusting (adjustment reactions are normal and expectable) impaired his learning.

Report from the Speech Therapist

If a child has a speech problem or has received help from a speech or language therapist in the past, a report from the speech therapist will be requested.

The nature of the speech or language problems that have been identified will be given, and the kind of progress being made will be stated. The speech therapist will also indicate how well the child attends and cooperates and how hard he works to correct his problems. Because the speech therapist works with the child individually or in a very small group, she may observe that he attends and works better for her than he does in his large regular class. This will give the team clues about the conditions under which the child can and will perform.

Medical and Physical or Occupational Therapy

Reports may be requested from medical specialists or other therapists if deemed appropriate and considered necessary. In most instances, however, parental reports of medical conditions, treatments, and special therapies suffice. This information makes the teacher and professional staff sensitive to what the child and family have had to endure and gives clues to both the psychological and physiological bases of learning and behavior difficulties.

Educational Testing

Tests of learning adequacy, learning potential, and learning skills (achievement) are given. These may be administered by the educational specialist or the psychologist.

Tests that relate to learning adequacy (other than mental tests that are given by the psychologist) are commonly called *perceptual* or *process tests*. These tests measure how well a child takes in, discriminates, understands, remembers, and is able to express (give back) what he sees and hears. His visual motor function—how well he can reproduce on paper (or in actions) things he sees—is another kind of perceptual process tested. These tests are commonly called *visual and auditory discrimination, visual and auditory comprehension, visual and auditory memory,* and the like. The idea is to determine a child's efficiency of learning through the visual channel (printed material), through the auditory channel (oral instruction), and through the visual-motor channel (writing, drawing, and making things).

Tests of learning potential are a newer concept than mental ability tests. They attempt to eliminate the factor of previous learning that all children may not have had. By requiring a child to solve a new task after being taught some preliminary strategies, a child's (potential) rate of learning may be estimated. These tests are controversial because they deviate from traditional approaches to assessing abilities (change is hard to accept); but also because they are not well understood by professionals, and their theoretical bases are not well established or accepted. However, I believe they will receive more attention in the future.

Individual tests of achievement in all aspects of reading, written skills, spelling, and math are a part of the evaluation. The teacher's report of achievement levels and the scores from group standardized tests are used for purposes of comparison. The aim is to determine at what level a child's skills are in relation to national norms as well as in relation to his classmates. Sometimes a child will prove to have skills well above what he shows himself to have in class. Sometimes a child can read words very well but cannot comprehend or remember well what he has read. The problem might prove to be that the child has average skills (national norms) but the level of the classroom instruction is well above average.

Psychological Testing

The most threatening aspect of the Child Study Evaluation is usually the psychological evaluation. The parent may fear that the child will reveal family secrets or that the child will be "pumped" about intimate family matters. Parents need more discussion and reassurance about this part of the evaluation than any other.

Usually, both ability tests (commonly referred to as IQ tests) and personality tests will be given. In the process of administering these tests, the psychologist hopes to deduce ideas about the child's learning style, his temperamental response to challenge and failure, his ability to function under time pressures, and his ability to work independently. Whether he has problems with self-esteem and whether anxiety disorganizes or immobilizes him will be other questions the psychologist hopes to answer. The goals are to find out whether the child has specific intellectual deficits that impede learning; whether he is a slow, average, or fast learner; what his attitudes toward achievement are (ideas about his motivation); and how well he is coping with conflicts and fears.

During the process of establishing rapport (which precedes the testing) the psychologist will interview the child in a fairly structured manner, asking him to express his positive and negative feelings about school, siblings, and friends. He will be asked questions about his worries, fears, hopes, and desires. Some children cannot tell things about themselves in such a direct way, and others will answer with what they are supposed to think and feel, rather than with their true feelings or their own thoughts. This is why the psychologist also uses other ways of eliciting a child's views.

A child conveys something of his inner self, his inner world, uncensored by his superego, in his drawings, his responses to ink blots, and in the stories he makes up. The psychologist asks a child to make up stories to go with pictures he is shown. These are called *projective techniques*. The child's feelings, attitudes, conflicts, and ways in which he copes will be reflected in his responses to this projective.

Intellectual functioning is assessed by administering a series of tasks of increasing difficulty that measure reasoning, judgment, spatial ability, abstract thinking, and so on. The child will be asked to tell what words mean, reason out problem situations, analyze and reconstruct patterns using blocks, put puzzles together, find what is missing in a picture, tell in what way two different objects or entities are alike, and so on. The tests are set up in such a way that the child will be asked some questions that are very easy and others that are so difficult he won't be expected to answer. It sometimes helps children to know this so they don't get the idea that they did poorly just because they couldn't answer some of the questions put to them.

COLLATING DATA FROM THE CHILD STUDY EVALUATION

When all the interviews and tests have been completed and relevant reports received, the special staff meets with the teacher to analyze and synthesize the data. The needs of the child are defined and recommendations decided upon. The recommendations will be presented to the parents at a subsequent meeting. Although the evaluation will usually have simultaneously answered all questions about a child, further evaluation of psychological problems or investigation of possible undiagnosed medical problems are occasionally among the conclusions of the study.

In analyzing the data gathered during a Child Study Evaluation, the staff will be viewing all the bits and pieces as a detective would. Inconsistencies and discrepancies will receive particular attention. Does the child who acts dull and uncomprehending in the classroom prove to have a low IQ, as expected, or does his IQ prove to be high? Does he show an adequate skill development on tests in contrast to his classroom performance, which is well below average? Is he able to read nonsense words well, thus demonstrating a very good grasp of phonics, but unable to read real words correctly? Is his oral reading comprehension poor while his silent reading comprehension above grade? Teachers are understandably surprised when a child proves to be a different child on the tests than he shows himself to be in the classroom, but this does happen. There are many times when the evaluation confirms most of the teacher's hypotheses about the child's learning problem. However, most frequently, the results comprise both surprises and validation of hunches.

TEACHER AND PARENT ROLES IN THE CHILD STUDY EVALUATION

Teachers initiate a Child Study Evaluation and are involved in the process from beginning to end. They recommend the evaluation, give parents information about it, and guide the parents through the process. They may be instrumental in obtaining parental permission when parents are at first resistant to the idea, by allaying parental fears. Parents also are involved in the evaluation at the outset and are expected to participate fully in the final conference when the conclusions of the study are presented to them.

Typically, when a child is having significant problems in school, the principal is informed and he evaluates whether a child study is indicated. There are things a principal may think should be done to try to remedy a problem before deciding on a referral for a Child Study Evaluation. For example, a trial period of counseling, outside tutoring, or a behavioral-motivational program supervised by the psychologist or counselor may be decided upon. When these efforts fail to bring the desired results, a meeting of all school staff who have been involved with the child may be held to determine other possible courses of action. At this point, it may be concluded that a Child Study Evaluation is necessary before further decisions are made.

If it is the consensus of the school staff that evaluation is necessary, the parents' signed permission for the evaluation must be obtained. If the teacher is the one expected to obtain parental permission, she should proceed in the manner described in the following section. In some schools, the principal or the counselor assumes the role of obtaining the parents' permission. In these instances, the request for permission may be only a formal procedure with the preparation of the parent by the teacher having taken place earlier.

The teacher begins to condition the parent for a proposed evaluation by stating very specifically what she needs to know about the child in order to help him learn. The evaluation can answer her questions. It can also determine whether the child qualifies for help from an educational specialist. She asks if the parent has any objections to such an evaluation. The parent will usually want to know exactly what goes on, what the evaluation consists of. The teacher then describes the components of the study, indicating what can be learned from each part. The teacher asks the mother to go home and talk with the father about what has been said (unless he has attended this conference). If there are further questions, they can be answered by phone or at a follow-up conference. If the parents agree to the evaluation, the teacher says that the counselor will soon call to set up an appointment. She then informs the counselor.

If the mother reports that she and father are uncertain or don't want to go ahead with the evaluation, the teacher asks for a **conference** to discuss it further. At this conference the teacher will want to discern the parents' fears that underlie their uncertainty or refusal. She should ask, "Can you tell me what makes you uncertain about agreeing to the evaluation?" or "I'm sorry you and your husband have decided not to let our staff do the evaluation. Can you tell me what your thoughts or feelings are that caused you to come to that decision?" The teacher should then just listen, not try to dispute or disqualify any of the reasons given, although explanations can be offered in response to fears expressed. A joint parental decision to refuse the evaluation will not be quickly reversed, and the teacher should not try to talk them out of their decision immediately. She should reaffirm her rationale for recommending the evaluation and tell the parents that she hopes they change their minds.

The situation is different if uncertainty exists. The parents are obviously ambivalent. They may need more information or they may need to have their fears allayed (see the following section). The teacher should respond by clarifying and reassuring. She should reiterate the value of doing the evaluation. She should then remain available to answer any new questions that may arise as they try to become comfortable with the idea of going ahead, of giving their approval for the evaluation.

PARENTAL FEARS

Many parents have a number of fears about having their child evaluated. For the most part, these seem to be based on incomplete information, false rumors, or incorrect generalizations.

One fear is that being referred for the evaluation is tantamount to saying that their child is either emotionally disturbed or retarded.

- Mrs. B's good friend has a child who is emotionally disturbed. She was told this on the basis of a psychological examination.

- Mrs. M has a retarded child. The psychologist did tests that showed this to be so.

The teacher should tell a parent that the evaluation *could* lead to conclusions about emotional disturbance or retardation. However, prejudgments are not appropriate, and more than a psychologist's test results go into the conclusion. Parents always participate in the process of evaluation and consideration of the results. For most children evaluated by a school staff, neither emotional disturbance nor mental retardation is the diagnosis. Most children either have learning disabilities or mild emotional difficulties.

Another fear held by some parents is that if their child is evaluated, he will be put into a special class. For some children, as already discussed, special class placement is desirable, and a Child Study Evaluation is a necessary step toward obtaining such a placement. However, a child cannot be placed in a special class without parental permission. The evaluation may qualify a child for a special class, but the parents have to agree to placement before this can come about. The teacher must make this clear to the parent.

A third fear commonly expressed is that the information from the evaluation retained in a child's record will bias others against him or exclude him from some opportunity in the future. This is a legitimate concern. However, safeguards for the parents and the child exist in the form of rights determined by the rules and regulations arising out of law. Parents have a right to know what is in the record, to request that statements be changed or deleted, and to request that reports be removed or destroyed when they are no longer relevant. Confidentiality is further maintained by keeping information from a Child Study Evaluation in a central office file, or only with the principal, counselor, or psychologist. The teacher should let the parents know what their rights are, refer them to an appropriate administrator to discuss this, or tell them that their rights are spelled out in a booklet the school has prepared for them (and be sure they have this). Many schools have prepared a booklet that is given to the parents. However, this should not replace the teacher's discussion of the whole procedure with the parent.

Another source of apprehension about the evaluation stems from the expectation that the child will be upset by the testing. This can make parents and sometimes even the teacher wary of having the evaluation, even when they objectively understand the reasons the testing is needed. In the case of a chronically ill child, they say "He has already been subjected to many examinations and treatments; why put him through more?" Experience suggests that children are not often upset by this procedure, although they may have questions, worries, or unfounded fears that need to be expressed. The child who has a brother or sister in a special class may be afraid the evaluation means that he will be put in a special class also. Even if the sibling of a special class child doesn't express this fear, it should be assumed that he is worried about this. He should be invited to say anything that is on his mind about it, and reassurance should be offered.

The child must be told why the evaluation is being done and what will be required of him. This is the parents' job, but the teacher (or counselor) will need to give the parent a general idea of what to say.

The child should also be told the names of the people he will meet with and what their jobs are in the school. It is a good idea to write this on a card for the child. The manner in which the parent and the teacher will participate should also be explained. The more information the child is given and the more open the parents are in talking about it, the more comfortable the child will be with the whole procedure (unless anxiety is transmitted in the discussions between the parents and the child). Children generally accept what they must do in school without becoming upset, even if this is different from what most other children have to do.

Children usually know when they are in trouble academically or behaviorally. In telling a child about the impending evaluation, the parent should start with a statement of fact; for example:

> You know you haven't been getting your work finished; you know your work hasn't been up to the teacher's expectations; you know you have been hitting other children.

It is important to be as clear and specific about his problem as possible.

The next statement is to convey that the testing procedure is to get information about his abilities, feelings, what he has already learned and remembered, and what he has missed out on learning. The teacher needs this kind of information to help him with his problem. The child should be encouraged to ask questions and express any feelings so the parents can offer reassurance or explanations. Reactions a child is likely to have pertain to worry over what will happen or how his parents will feel if he doesn't do well on the tests, what his friends will think or say, and what he might be missing in class during the time he is being tested. It is important to schedule testing so that field trips, sport events, or any other special school or family events are not missed.

This was somewhat overlooked in Raymond's case, but he was bold enough to assert himself with the examiner.

> Raymond, the star of the seventh grade soccer team, told the examiner he had to be finished by 2:30 in order to be back at school in time for an important soccer game. (He was being tested in a central office.) The examiner made sure that he was out on time (the testing usually lasted until 3:00).

In Margaret's case, it was important that she expressed her fears before the testing took place.

Margaret was afraid that being tested meant she would be put in a special class (she had a friend who had been tested and then went to a special class). Her mother told her she was sure this wouldn't happen. Then her mother mentioned it to the psychologist, who also reassured Margaret (although testing can lead to special class placement, the indications that this is *not* likely to be an outcome are usually evident beforehand).

Ted's worry was about how his parents felt about him.

Ted thought his parents were angry at him for needing to be tested because he knew they were upset about his low scores on weekly tests and his failure to finish his assignments. Ted's mother told him she *had* been angry at his poor schoolwork, but maybe she had been wrong; maybe he had a special problem with learning that the tests could shed some light on. If that were the case, he could get some help, and his parents could become more understanding.

Children of school age should be told about the evaluation a week ahead of the appointment time. They need time to think of questions, to express worries, and to assimilate the fact that the testing is an effort to find a solution to their problems. If a mother is afraid that her child will react negatively and resist going for the appointment, she may be tempted to delay telling him until it is time to go for the appointment. However, this is very unwise. The school-age child will feel resentful toward his mother for springing the news on him, and he is likely to act rebellious with the examiners. Some rebellious children may show their anger by giving wrong answers, or their feelings of anger may subconsciously impair their functioning. Either reaction can lead to invalid test results. A parent who does not tell her child that he has a testing appointment until the morning of the appointment or the night before is treating him like a very young child.

Sometimes an evaluation of abilities, skills, and personality has been done outside the school, in a hospital or community health center, for example. The parents will usually expect the school to accept a report of that evaluation as a substitute for a proposed school evaluation. However, the school staff may consider the outside evaluation to be incomplete or may consider the recommendations from it unrealistic. The report of the outside evaluation may be filled with psychological jargon and may not convey a meaningful picture of the child. In explaining to the parent the need for a Child Study Evaluation to be done at school, it is wise *not* to criticize the outside evaluation. "Incompleteness," "lack of specificity," or the "basis for the recommendations not stated" are explanations that can be given in a matter-of-fact manner, without criticizing the other evaluation. It is important to use diplomacy; the parent may be exasperated, having had the outside evaluation done with the understanding that it would answer the questions being raised about her child.

The Child Study Evaluation and implementation of the recommendations that emerge from it require a team effort. The team consists of teachers, parents, and a number of professionals. Experience has shown that it takes a lot of new learning of interpersonal skills to achieve satisfactory team functioning.

In Chapter 10, I discussed some of the skills that are necessary to overcome barriers between teachers and parents, and between doctors and teachers. In the final chapter, I analyze in more detail the reasons it has been so difficult for teachers, parents, and other professionals to work together effectively. Awareness is the starting point of change. The ultimate goal is for teachers to become partners with parents and other professionals in order to serve the best interests of children.

13

TEACHERS AS PARTNERS WITH PARENTS AND OTHER PROFESSIONALS

> Ellen has a busy schedule for a nine-year-old: On Tuesdays and Saturdays she goes to her allergist for desensitization shots; Wednesdays are family therapy meetings; she has Mrs. Tate for tutoring on Mondays and Fridays; and on Thursdays she goes to the hospital for Group with other children who have bad asthma. She visits her pediatrician often because of frequent headaches and stomachaches.

The future can be brighter for children like Ellen if the many professionals they are involved with work together harmoniously. All adults in an ill child's life, as well as the parents, are authority figures, models by which the child shapes her thinking and behavior. What kinds of models do the adults present? Do they find fault, criticize, and get angry at each other? Do they model cooperation, mutual respect, and complementarity of roles? The latter requires teamwork.

In order to work together in cooperative team fashion, adults must feel that they have equal status with each other. Recognition of this basic premise immediately poses a dilemma as it is contrary to the hierarchical structures on which our culturally conditioned patterns of behavior have been established. Status positions have traditionally defined the nature of relationships between people as "up-down." In the status structure, the doctor has historically held the most "up" position. In a doctor-teacher or doctor-parent encounter, the doctor would expect to be dominant/superior; the teacher or parent, submissive/inferior. Between teacher and parent, the teacher would expect to have the "up" position. These status positions are deeply ingrained. It is only since the team concept has become a popular model for working out solutions to difficult problems that the necessity for changing these status patterns of relating has become apparent.

If teacher, doctor, and parents are to have equal status regarding relating to each other, old patterns of relating in a dominant-submissive way must be relinquished. (For clarity of discussion, all school professionals will be subsumed as teacher and all medical and mental health professionals outside the school will be subsumed as doctor.)

Parents are the real experts on their own child; they know him best. They must feel confident about asserting themselves with the doctor and the teacher. The doctor does not have to act superior toward the parents and the teacher in order to assure that his medical orders will be followed. He must feel secure that the parents and the teacher respect his medical authority, even though they may assert themselves with him about psychological and educational issues. The teacher has a mandate to educate but does not have to be intimidating in relating to parents. The teacher should not assume a down position role, as if she is on the inferior side of a superior-inferior relationship pattern in conferring with a student's doctor. Parents, teachers, and doctors must accord each other respect. They should each expect to be listened to with genuine regard as they voice their individual concerns about a child.

ROLES, RESPONSIBILITIES, REALITIES

Typically, parents, doctors, and teachers, in trying to work together, have encountered problems. One or more of these reasons may be contributory: blurred understanding of roles, communication breakdowns regarding responsibilities, and individual realities, precipitating reactions that are often misunderstood by others. These difficulties—clarifying roles, assigning responsibilities, and understanding the realities of each other's situation—can result in angry feelings, which in turn lead to negative interacting. Blaming replaces responsible action. A doctor gets upset at a parent for not carrying out the medical regimen or for making unreasonable demands. Parents project their pent-up frustrations onto the teacher or the doctor. The teacher is insulted if the doctor makes an educational recommendation. The doctor jumps to erroneous conclusions on the basis of slanted reports from the parent or the child and starts to believe that the teacher is acting in a prejudicial or nonprofessional manner. Whatever the basis for negative judgments, it is far too easy (and common) for the child's important adults to distance themselves from each other. Instead of trying to correct misunderstandings, see the other's point of view, make compromises, and give each other support in the difficult task each is trying to accomplish with the child, they unwittingly create barriers.

Roles

Once it has been agreed that there is a joint responsibility between parents, doctors, and teachers for the child's rearing and schooling, the first task is to clarify the boundaries of each person's role. Keeping the child as well and healthy as possible must take priority, and all have a role in this. The doctor must provide the leadership in clarifying what is expected from the parent and the teacher (and also the child) in terms of each one's role in health care. The doctor's role is to supervise the child's health care, and the teacher's and parent's roles are to carry out his directives. The doctor must tell the parent and the teacher what to do and what not to do; specify for them the symptoms that would necessitate a call to the doctor; and instruct them as to how to deal with a potential medical emergency. He should be willing to answer questions put to him by the teacher or the parent as each of these important adults tries to understand the basic mechanisms of the illness. He should try to help his child patient understand his illness to the degree that his emerging cognitive abilities allow and as he matures, teach him self-care.

The moral, social, and emotional development of the child is primarily the parents' domain, but the teacher and the doctor have a part to play. It has already been outlined how the doctor and the teacher help a child grow. They have important contributions to make in a child's development, and the parents are usually grateful. If the parents are confused or disapproving of the doctor's or the teacher's efforts, it is important to work out the disagreements. The parents feel strongly that their child's overall development is their domain and that the efforts of doctor and teacher must fit in with their value system. If a child is not developing as well as is desirable (and possible), from the doctor's or the teacher's point of view, they must try to decide with the parents what should be done.

Parents are sometimes resistant to the idea that they or their child need counseling. However, they are usually receptive to the insights offered by professionals. Teachers may suggest counseling, but a doctor or psychologist making such a recommendation can carry more weight with parents. Teachers should not feel offended if parents do not accept such a recommendation from them but are willing to follow through when they are told the same thing by a doctor, psychologist, (or both). The important goal is to get help for the child and his family.

It is always wise for the teacher to consult with the doctor from the outset when there are indications that counseling is needed. In guiding parents toward counseling, parental decision-making power must be respected. The doctor and the teacher must help a family accept the idea of counseling and guide them to services available.

The teacher has the major role in teaching a child academic skills. She also must stimulate and nurture his intellect. The parents and the doctor aid the teacher in achieving her purpose by their roles in fostering motivation. They must help the child *want* to be in school and *want* to make the effort to learn. They must help him with his feelings about his illness or physical handicap. They must give him appropriate instruction about what to do if he develops symptoms in school so he will feel safe being there away from home or hospital. They will need to rehearse with him ways to answer the questions, curiosity, or teasing of children who can be expected to react to the physical or medical things that mark him as different.

It is easy to say that a doctor's role is to cure, a parent's role is to rear, and a teacher's role is to educate. But what does it mean? Parents also educate. Doctors know they can't cure in many instances, but they also educate in a variety of ways. Teachers nurture, discipline, help children socialize, and also contribute to moral development, all of which are part of the rearing role. These are the reasons that role boundaries can become blurred.

Role Boundary Difficulties

Parents must maintain positive regard and a warm, sensitive rapport with their child if their rearing efforts are to be effective. They usually want to be helpful to their child in every way possible. There is a strong tendency on the teacher's part, when a child is having trouble in school, to ask the parents to help him at home. Parents will be cooperative and start working with the child on math, reading, or other subjects. When they take on the tutoring job, they become coercive and judgmental with their child regarding his school assignments. The child then reacts with resistance and anger, and parents become frustrated and upset. This turns a positive parent-child relationship into a negative one. It is the teacher's job to judge the child's efforts. Parents must not be asked to be academic tutors to their own child, but it is appropriate for the teacher to ask the parent to be sure that homework is completed and returned. If the work is poorly done, or incorrect, the teacher will judge it and point out errors to the child.

A teacher's role is to maintain control of a group of children for the purpose of conducting a class and delivering instruction. It is not appropriate for a parent to dictate how this should be accomplished. A teacher's realities may allow some actions and disallow others. The teacher can be spontaneous and creative only within certain limits. A parent who expects her child to be treated in the same way that he is treated at home is not being understanding of a teacher's reality. It is also possible that the teacher, seeing a child more objectively than parents can, knows that the child will benefit from having to adjust to a different reality than he has at home.

The doctor's primary role is the medical management of the child's illness. This requires the cooperation of the parents and the teacher. The doctor is not always there; he depends on the other adults to see that his recommendations are carried out. He must be sure his instructions are understood. In the process of conveying instructions, he may also offer helpful hints (guidance). There may be some leeway for parental decision making. He must clearly differentiate between what is essential regarding care and what is optional. Some doctors expect their guidance to be adhered to as strictly as their orders; this is not the way guidance is perceived by others. Teachers must ask doctors to be very specific about what is essential and what is optional. Parents also understand that guidance is optional and intuitively know that some suggestions do not fit their situation. They will usually seek to be reassured that noncompliance in such instances will not make the doctor disagreeable toward them or their child.

A doctor may insist that a child should have as normal a life as possible, which to him means that the child should be in a regular class at school. This may not be at all realistic from the school's point of view. On the other hand, the doctor may feel that a child needs a special class when the school staff in charge of making such decisions cannot justify such a placement. In these instances, doctors are overstepping the boundaries of their role and responsibility and creating situations of conflict that cause difficulty for school personnel.

A mother may press a doctor to excuse her child from gym when he feels that the physical education program is of benefit to the child. A parent may press a teacher to provide homework when the teacher sees this as unwise. These are ways in which parents overstep their boundaries and create dilemmas for doctors or teachers.

A teacher may advise that a child should see a neurologist or take pills for his hyperactivity. A teacher may presume to tell a parent how to discipline her child or require that the parent work with the child on academics. These are ways in which teachers overstep their boundaries.

Responsibilities

The primary responsibility of each adult, be it parent or professional, is to make sure that his role boundaries are not invaded. This requires that each clarify for the other when he feels his boundary is being overstepped. For boundary clarification to take place, each adult must be assertive. This is why equal status in relating is so necessary. It is difficult to be assertive if a person feels himself to be in a down or inferior status position. When a person is being assertive about what he perceives as his proper role, he is in effect criticizing or challenging another's words or actions. The other may become defensive. The boundary defender can either back down or stick to his position. The decision about which is correct to do depends on the arguments raised by the other. It is possible that in differences of opinion, there can be two rights and no wrongs.

When roles have been clearly defined with boundary issues clarified, parents and professional participants should each know what their responsibilities are. The problem, though, is in communication. In order for boundary problems to be clarified, communication must be kept open and meanings clearly understood. Communication breakdowns occur for various reasons, and when this happens, efforts must be made to reestablish rapport. Sometimes this requires intervention from outside.

The following case illustrates how an outside agency can be used effectively when communication has broken down between teacher and parents, and between doctor and parents:

> The Browns were a young couple whose first child, born when they were twenty, was diagnosed as having infantile spasms when he was nine months old. This kind of seizure, typically associated with mental retardation and behavior disorder, is hard to control. Mrs. Brown became greatly distressed in rearing this baby boy who fell forward with a stiff jerk at frequent intervals. At age seven, the parents brought Mike to a multi-disciplinary hospital clinic. Mike had a very confused history that included several kinds of seizures and alternating periods when his doctor thought he did not have seizures, but rather a behavior disorder. He had been on and off many kinds of medications. The school suspected that Mike was retarded, but his parents had refused to allow the school to test him. The parents were extremely angry and upset. The evaluation done by the clinic proved that Mike was not retarded; he had low-average mental ability and a learning disability. He clearly had epilepsy. He needed to be in a special class because of the complex nature

of his disability. His seizures were poorly controlled, he had difficulty learning, and his behavior could become erratic. However, he did not do well, even in the special class, and now the parental anxiety became severe. Both the doctor and the teacher received so many anxious, upset, angry phone calls from the parents that they felt they could no longer be helpful to them. The phone calls were either very demanding or very confusing in angry accusations. The teacher and the doctor agreed that the family should be referred back to the hospital clinic. In order to get the situation under control, several ground rules were established. The clinic staff was to serve as advocate, counselor, and liaison between the parents and the doctor, and the parents and the school. All messages from the family were to be channeled through the clinic. The clinic's pediatrician would call the child's doctor if there were questions or confusions about medication. The clinic's psychologist began counseling the mother and was the contact person between her and the school. Counseling restored the mother's self-esteem, taught her how to deal with anxiety, instructed her about school laws and parental rights, helped her to see what the teacher's and the doctor's realities were, and helped her improve her communication skills. She and the counselor rehearsed and role-played ways to talk to school staff. Ultimately, Mrs. Brown was able to relate in a cooperative, respectful way with both the teacher and the doctor.

The clinic staff was effective in restoring rapport between this family and the school, and between them and their doctor because the clinic was in a neutral position. The clinic had gained this neutrality for several reasons: They did not have to deal with the day-to-day issues that the teacher and the doctor had with the family; they were held in high regard by the parents because of the clinic's role (and support) in clarifying Mike's problems; and the staff were all experienced in working with teachers and doctors (many had previously worked in schools and, of course, currently worked with doctors), and had high respect for them.

Clear understanding of responsibilities allows each participant to resist taking on too much, becoming overly responsible. It also permits each to feel that he is doing his part. Most important, it helps each one to recognize where and how he must hold the others accountable for their parts.

Mrs. R. felt that she must help her daughter do better in school. She insisted that Jane read to her every night. She checked her written reports and made her copy them over if they were sloppily done. She quizzed her on spelling and made her work on math problems even when the teacher had not given homework. Her previously pleasant relationship with Jane soon became a nightmare of angry recriminations. The tension between mother and Jane had become almost intolerable. When the teacher and counselor told the mother to stop working with Jane, the mother felt immediately relieved. She did not really want the job of helping her daughter do better but had considered it her parental responsibility to do so.

Mrs. R. learned that it was not her responsibility to improve her daughter's academic skills. In the future, she would be able to resist a teacher's expectations that she tutor or judge her daughter's schoolwork.

Realities

Parents, doctor, and teachers have different realities. Realities are the particular difficulties, dilemmas, and pressures that adults experience within their own sphere. Realities include the rules that govern what a parent or professional can and cannot do. Realities encompass such things as how many patients a doctor has, how many students a teacher has, and whether or not each one has adequate help and support. The amount of power that one has to control events is a most important factor in each one's reality situation. It is important that doctors, teachers, and parents know each other's realities and be sensitive to them.

It is possible to talk about realities in general; that is, to be aware that teachers must adhere to the rules stipulated by law and implemented by the policies of the local school board. They must cover the curriculum stipulated, aim to keep all children up to grade level (whether or not this is possible), keep the children safe, and so on. They are subject to censure for the way they talk, the manner in which they conduct their classes, and sometimes even for the way they live their private lives. They are held accountable by the threat of dismissal and the withholding of tenure.

Doctors are governed by the ethics of their profession, licensure by the state, which may stipulate what they can and cannot do, and by the rules and regulations of the hospital with which they are associated. They are held accountable by threat of malpractice suits and loss of licensure for misconduct.

Parents are obligated to rear their children in keeping with the implicit standards of the culture. When the culture is diverse, as it is in the United States, there is considerable latitude and a range of patterns that is acceptable. Parents also are held accountable. They must not abuse their children. They must send them to school, and they must strive to feed, clothe, and keep them healthy to the best of their ability.

Within this framework of general realities, a particular doctor, teacher, or set of parents has a specific reality. There is only one way for anyone else to be able to appreciate the pressures or dilemmas of that specific reality. It must be communicated. If parents feel pressured by economic difficulties, they can let the doctor or the teacher know. If the doctor feels that her integrity is compromised by certain demands of a patient or hospital board, she cannot give the exact reason, but she may be able to convey to others that she is under pressure. The teacher may be in serious disagreement with the strictures of the school board and feel that he can do little about the matter. It would be very difficult and probably unwise for him to openly express this, but he may be able to get across the idea that he wishes things could work differently. Perhaps he could ask the parents if they agree with the school board's policies, and if they do not, to encourage them to take a stand.

The first step in regard to realities is to be aware of them as a factor affecting the way a person reacts. If negative interactions are occurring, it could be helpful to think about what might be going on in the other person's reality situation. A reality that is common to all, for example, is frustration. The doctor can become quite upset and frustrated, simply because she is powerless to make a patient better—and in the case of degenerative disorders, she simply can't. The teacher feels the same kind of frustration when he has a slow-learning child who can't grasp what he is teaching. What about the parents who do everything the doctor says and the capricious illness gets out of control anyway? Once reality factors are acknowledged as a source of tension, it is possible for understanding and effective relating to replace conflict. A person can either try to change realities or exert his energies toward working around them.

SUMMING UP

Although professionals and researchers have increasingly become knowledgeable about the needs of the chronically ill child and his family, the general public lacks awareness and understanding. Despite the gains that have been made in providing for the needs of the chronically ill child, there is a long way to go in lessening the tremendous burden for him and his family. There are still many children who get inadequate medical care, many families enormously strained by the financial burden and psychological stress, far too many unenlightened professionals, and too few sources of support and help. However, there is optimism for the future.

A major study entitled "Public Policies Affecting Chronically Ill Children and Their Families" has been completed at Vanderbilt University's Institute for Public Policy Studies. The findings of the study have been published as *Chronically Ill Children and Their Families: Today's Challenge for Health and Education* (Jossey-Bass, San Francisco, 1985).

The aim of the final report will be to develop the public's awareness of the special needs of children with severe chronic illnesses. The hope is that these needs will be more adequately provided for by responsible societal action once public awareness is aroused. The project has identified issues and problems in the organization and financing of medical and nonmedical services, in policies and programs of the schools and community, and in research and training programs.

The Vanderbilt project's findings regarding the schools confirm the significance of the issues discussed in this book. Additional concerns are disclosed by the study, which have not been dealt with here. They center around medical care needed during school attendance and the limited health services available in schools, the need for more flexible policies regarding homebound and hospital instruction, the need for children to receive "related services" as defined by PL 94-142 regardless of needing "special education," and the need of some chronically ill children for specialized instruction (in areas related to their medical and physical condition) in addition to the regular curriculum.* Until these issues have been dealt with, the tasks for the teacher, as discussed throughout this book, will not be so easily accomplished. The teacher can know that she is a pioneer in this important sphere, and that her efforts will contribute toward full societal awareness.

The needs of the chronically ill child and the challenges he and his family must face change in tandem with the illness and the child's own development. As the child gets better, he picks up the threads of normal development. He needs time to fill in the gaps and to make up for what was lost while he was ill. He will progress along the normal developmental lines, but he may have trouble catching up to what is

---

*Adapted from *Chronically Ill Children and Their Families: Today's Challenge for Health and Education* by Nicholas Hobbs, James M. Perrin, and Henry T. Ireys, Jossey-Bass, San Francisco, 1985. Permission given by James M. Perrin.

expected of a child his age. Parents and teachers should appreciate the effort he makes to catch up and the time it takes. They must realize that if the child views the task of catching up as too overwhelming, he will not want to make the effort. He will be pulled in the direction of regression, of resisting growing up.

I have shown the teacher how to help, to ensure that the child will keep moving in the direction of growth. Until parents become fully knowledgeable, teachers should guide them toward services within the school and within the community.

Parents may deplete their psychic and physical energies during the many years of coping with their child's illness. Periodically they need breathing space and time for renewal. When they have completed the long journey through the childhood crises, they may begin to feel some freedom. The chronically ill adolescent and young adult still needs her parents; but the child grown up insists on carrying the burden of making decisions about her treatment and of handling the emotional impact of the illness on her own. As the grown-up child assumes increasing responsibility for herself, the parents have more time. As bodies become rested and spirits refreshed, many parents begin to want to do something for others who must go through what they have. Parents who have graduated from their caretaking role and recovered their energy will find a wide range of activities needing workers or leaders.

If there is no program in their community for helping the families of chronically ill children (as described in Chapter 9), energized parents may want to get a program started. If programs are available, they may want to become volunteers. Volunteers are also needed in hospital child-life programs and in schools. Libraries need more books on the subjects of illness, hospitalization, self-help groups, and coping. Legislation is needed for mandating and financing the many services required by the ill child and his family. Camping, recreational, and social programs are needed that will meet the special requirements of ill children. Special education legislation must be maintained. Medical research must be supported. Lobbying, fund raising, giving time to human services or to community education and awareness are among the activities that parents may wish to become involved in.

Societal goals regarding health education and quality of life are implicit in the actions and purposes of many public and private organizations. They are also stated in federal and state laws and in the regulations that govern implementation of such legislation. Here are a few that are relevant:

- To provide good medical care to all
- To maximize psychosocial support for ill and hospitalized children and their families
- To promote and support research that will reduce suffering from illness and disability to the greatest degree possible
- To assure that every child, regardless of health impairment or physical handicap, has the opportunity to develop to his full potential both intellectually and socially
- To keep children in the mainstream to the extent that is feasible.

Teachers and other school personnel join the many important adults in a child's life to help him cope and grow. When teachers become partners with parents and other professionals and embrace these goals, they share the responsibility for his rearing, schooling, and medical care. By sharing the responsibility, the tremendous task involved becomes less overwhelming and of more reasonable proportion to all involved.

BIBLIOGRAPHY

BOOKS FOR CHILDREN

About Illness (younger children)

Baker, Lynn S., *You and Leukemia: A Day at a Time*. Philadelphia: W. B. Saunders, 1978.

Fassler, Joan, *Howie Helps Himself*. Chicago: Albert Whitman, 1975. About a child with cerebral palsy.

Jones, Rebecca C., *Angie and Me*. New York: Macmillan, 1981. About a child with arthritis.

Silverstein, Alvin and Virginia Silverstein, *Itch, Sniffle, and Sneeze: All about Asthma, Hay Fever, and Other Allergies*. Englewood Cliffs, NJ: Scholastic Book Service, 1978.

There Is a Rainbow Behind Every Dark Cloud. Millbrae, CA: Celestial Arts, 1978. A book of children's drawings depicting their inner experiences of serious illness, struggle for survival, and worry about death.

About Illness (children nine and older)

Biklen, Douglas and Michell Sokoloff, *What Do You Do When Your Wheelchair Gets a Flat Tire?* Englewood Cliffs, NJ: Scholastic Book Service, 1978. Questions and answers about a variety of disabilities, asked by normal children and answered by disabled children.

Blume, Judy, *Deenie*. New York: Dell, 1974. About a girl with scoliosis.

Jones, Ron, *The Acorn People*. New York: Bantam, 1977. About physically handicapped children at camp.

Silverstein, Alvin and Virginia Silverstein, *Epilepsy*. New York: Harper and Row, 1975.

———*Run Away Sugar: All about Diabetes*. New York: Harper and Row, 1981.

Singer, Marilyn, *It Can't Hurt Forever*. New York: Harper and Row, 1978. About a girl who has a heart operation.

Slote, Alfred, *Hang Tough, Paul Mather*. Philadelphia: J. B. Lippincott, 1973. About a boy who has leukemia.

Southall, Ivan, *Let the Balloon Go*. London: Penguin Books, 1968. About an overly protected boy who has cerebral palsy.

About Hospitalization

Bemelmans, Ludwig, *Madeline*. New York: Viking Press, 1967.

Howe, James, *The Hospital Book*. New York: Crown, 1981.

Livingston, Carole and Claire Ciliotta, *Why Am I Going to the Hospital?* Secaucus, NJ: Lyle Stuart, 1981.

Rey, Margaret and H. A. Rey, *Curious George Goes to the Hospital*. Boston: Houghton Mifflin, 1966.

Shay, Arthur, *What Happens When You Go to the Hospital?* Chicago: Reilly and Lee, 1969.

Stein, Sara B., *A Hospital Story*. New York: Walker, 1974.

Tambourine, Jean, *I Think I Will Go to the Hospital*. Nashville, TN: Abingdon Press, 1965.

About Siblings' Reactions

Baznik, Donna, *Becky's Story*. Washington, DC: Association for the Care of Children's Health, 1981. A book for siblings of hospitalized children.

Lasker, Joe, *He's My Brother*. Chicago: Albert Whitman, 1974. A young boy describes the home and school experiences of his younger brother who has a learning disability.

Lowry, Lois, *A Summer to Die*. New York: Bantam Books, 1979. About sisters, one of whom becomes terminally ill.

Straight from the Siblings: Another Look at the Rainbow. Millbrae, CA: Celestial Arts, 1982. Written by siblings of children who have life-threatening illnesses; includes the children's drawings as well as their stories.

Weber, Alfons, *Elizabeth Gets Well*. New York: Thomas Y. Crowell, 1970. Siblings' reactions when their sister has an operation.

About Death and Dying (younger children)

Lee, Virginia, *The Magic Moth*. New York: Seabury Press, 1972. A butterfly becomes a symbol of hope, and the funeral process is explained.

Smith, Doris, *A Taste of Blackberries*. New York: Thomas Y. Crowell, 1973. A boy comes to terms with the death of a friend.

About Death and Dying (children nine and older)

Carlson, Natalie, *The Half Sisters*. New York: Harper and Row, 1970. A girl copes with the death of a sister.

Corely, Elizabeth, *Tell Me about Death, Tell Me about Funerals*. Santa Clara, CA: Grammatical Sciences, 1973.

Ipswitch, E. *Scott Was Here*. New York: Dell, 1978. About a boy who dies of Hodgkin's disease.

Watts, Richard, *Straight Talk about Death with Young People*. Philadelphia: Westminster Press, 1975.

White, E. B., *Charlotte's Web*. New York: Harper and Row, 1952. This classic about anthropomorphized spider Charlotte is a favorite of dying children, who gain comfort from it. It can also be comforting to friends of a child who dies.

Zim, Herbert and Sonia Bleeker, *Life and Death*. New York: William Morrow, 1970. The book gives a survey of life functions, medical tests, and so forth.

BOOKS FOR PARENTS

A Child Goes to the Hospital (pamphlet). Washington, DC: Association for the Care of Children's Health, 1981.

Azarnoff, Pat and Carol Hardgrove, *The Family in Child Health Care*. New York: John Wiley and Sons, 1981.

Bank, Stephen P. and Michael D. Kahn, *The Sibling Bond*. New York: Basic Books, 1982.

Berger, Eugenia H., *Parents as Partners in Education*. St. Louis: C. V. Mosby, 1981.

Bluebond-Langner, Myra, *The Private Worlds of Dying Children*. Princeton, NJ: Princeton University Press, 1978.

Burns, David, *Feeling Good: The New Mood Therapy*. New York: William Morrow, 1980. A self-help guide for overcoming depression.

Bush, Richard, *When a Child Needs Help: A Parents' Guide to Child Therapy*. New York: Delacorte Press, 1980.

DeRosis, Helen A., *Women and Anxiety: A Step-by-Step Program for Managing Anxiety and Depression*. New York: Delacorte Press, 1979.

Fassler, Joan, *Helping Children Cope: Mastering Stress through Books and Stories*. New York: The Free Press, 1978.

Featherstone, Helen, *A Difference in the Family: Life with a Disabled Child.* New York: Basic Books, 1980.

Gordon, Audrey K. and Dennis Klass, *They Need to Know: How to Teach Children about Death.* Englewood Cliffs, NJ: Prentice-Hall, 1979.

Hobbs, Nicholas and James M. Perrin and Henry T. Ireys, *Chronically Ill Children and Their Families: Today's Challenge for Health and Education.* San Francisco: Jossey-Bass, 1985.

How to Get Services by Being Assertive. Chicago: Coordinating Council for Handicapped Children, 1980.

Koocher, Gerald P. and John E. O'Malley, *The Damocles Syndrome: Psychosocial Consequences of Surviving Childhood Cancer.* New York: McGraw-Hill, 1981.

Kübler-Ross, Elisabeth, *Living with Death and Dying.* New York: Macmillan, 1981.

_____*On Children and Death.* New York: Macmillan, 1983.

Lagos, Jorge, *Seizures, Epilepsy, and Your Child: A Handbook for Parents, Teachers, and Epileptics of All Ages.* New York: Harper and Row, 1974.

McCollum, Audrey, *The Chronically Ill Child: A Guide for Parents and Professionals.* New Haven, CT: Yale University Press, 1981.

Petrillo, Madeline and Sirgay Sanger, *Emotional Care of Hospitalized Children,* 2nd ed. New York: Harper and Row, 1980.

Pizzo, Peggy, *Parent to Parent: Working Together for Ourselves and Our Children.* Boston: Beacon Press, 1983.

Preparing Your Child for Repeated or Extended Hospitalizations (pamphlet). Washington, DC: Association for the Care of Children's Health, 1982.

Schaefer, Charles, ed., *Therapeutic Use of Child's Play.* New York: Jason Aronson, 1976.

Schiff, Harriet, *The Bereaved Parent.* New York: Penguin Books, 1978.

The Chronically Ill Child and Family in the Community (pamphlet). Washington, DC: Association for the Care of Children's Health, 1982.

Turnbull, Ann and H. Turnbull, *Parents Speak Out: Growing with a Handicapped Child.* Columbus, OH: Charles Merrill, 1979.

BOOKS FOR TEACHERS

A Child Goes to the Hospital and *A Guide for Teachers: Children and Hospitals* (pamphlets). Washington, DC: Association for the Care of. Children's Health, 1981.

Arnold, Eugene, ed., *Helping Parents Help Their Children.* New York: Brunner/Mazel, 1978.

Arnold, Joan and Penelope Gemma, *A Child Dies: A Portrait of Family Grief.* Rockville, MD: Aspen Systems, 1983.

Baskin, Barbara and Karen Harris, *Notes from a Different Drummer: A Guide to Juvenile Fiction Portraying the Handicapped.* New York: R. R. Bowker, 1977.

Bibace, Roger and Mary E. Walsh, eds., *Children's Conceptions of Health, Illness, and Bodily Functions.* San Francisco: Jossey-Bass, 1981.

Bleck, Eugene E. and Donald A. Nagel, eds., *Physically Handicapped Children: A Medical Atlas for Teachers,* 2nd ed. New York: Grune and Stratton, 1982.

Bloom, Benjamin, *All Our Children Learning.* New York: McGraw-Hill, 1981.

Buckley, Nancy K. and Hill M. Walker, *Modifying Classroom Behavior.* Champaign, IL: Research Press, 1978.

Farnham-Diggory, Sylvia, *Learning Disabilities.* Cambridge, MA: Harvard University Press, 1978.

Haslam, Robert and Peter Valletutti, eds., *Medical Problems in the Classroom: The Teacher's Role in Diagnosis and Management.* Baltimore: University Park Press, 1975.

Homme, Lloyd and others, *How to Use Contingency Contracting in the Classroom.* Champaign, IL: Research Press, 1970.

Kleinberg, Susan, *Educating the Chronically Ill Child.* Rockville, MD: Aspen Systems, 1982. This book, about continuity of education for the hospitalized child focuses on the role of the home and hospital teacher, provides medical information, and advises what appropriate approaches to take with the hospitalized child.

Kroth, Roger, *Communicating with Parents of Exceptional Children: Improving Parent-Teacher Relationships.* Denver, CO: Love Publishing, 1975.

McWhirter, J. Jeffries, *The Learning-Disabled Child.* Champaign, IL: Research Press, 1977.

Mullins, Jane, *A Teacher's Guide to Management of Physically Handicapped Students.* Springfield, IL: Charles Thomas, 1979.

Orlick, Terry, *The Cooperative Sports and Games Book: Challenge Without Competition.* New York: Pantheon Books, 1978.

Paul, James, ed., *Understanding and Working With Parents of Children with Special Needs.* New York: Holt, Rinehart and Winston, 1980.

Schaefer, Charles and Howard Millman, eds., *Therapies for Children: A Hand-*

book of Effective Treatments for Problem Behaviors. San Francisco: Jossey-Bass, 1977.

Schultz, Edward and Charles M. Heuchert, *Child Stress and the School Experience.* New York: Human Sciences Press, 1983.

Stephens, Thomas M., and Joan Wolf, *Effective Skills in Parent/Teacher Conferencing.* Columbus, OH: The National Center, Educational Media and Materials for the Handicapped/Ohio State University, 1980.

Swift, Marshall S. and George Spivak, *Alternate Teaching Strategies.* Champaign, IL: Research Press, 1975.

Travis, Georgia, *Chronic Illness in Children: Its Impact on Child and Family.* Stanford, CA: Stanford University Press, 1976.

Turnbull, Ann and Jane Schulz, *Mainstreaming Handicapped Students: A Guide for the Classroom Teacher.* Boston: Allyn and Bacon, 1979.

CURRICULUM GUIDES AND MATERIALS

Teaching About Death

They Need to Know: How to Teach Children About Death, by Audrey Gordon and Dennis Klass, Prentice-Hall, Englewood Cliffs, NJ 07632. A complete guide for grades kindergarten through high school.

Teaching About Individual Differences and Handicaps

Accepting Individual Differences, Developmental Learning Materials, 7440 Natchez Ave., Niles, IL. 60648. Kit for grades K–6.

Feeling Free (16mm film or videocassettes), Scholastic Book Service, 904 Sylvan Ave., Englewood Cliffs, NJ 07632. Each of five films introduces an engaging child who happens to be disabled in some way. Classroom readings, activities, and discussion materials are also available to complement the films.

Mainstreaming: What Every Child Needs to Know About Disabilities, by Susan Bookbinder. The Exceptional Parent Bookstore, 296 Boylston St., Boston, MA 02116. A discussion program that can be presented by trained volunteers, as well as by the classroom teacher.

People Just Like You: About Handicaps and Handicapped People. Superintendent of Public Documents, U.S. Government Printing Office, Washington, DC 20402 (stock number 040-000-00405-0). An activity guide for grades K–12.

Special Friends, Listen and Learn Company, 13366 Pescadero Rd., LaHonda, CA 94020. Kit suitable for grades K–3.

What Is a Handicap? BEA Educational Media, 2211 Michigan Ave., Santa Monica, CA 90404. Kit suitable for grades 4–6.

Teaching About Illness and Hospitalization

A Guide for Teachers: Children and Hospitals. Association for the Care of Children's Health, 3615 Wisconsin Ave. N.W., Washington, DC 20016. This inexpensive pamphlet presents concepts to teach, activities to have available, and a reading list.

Having an Operation, Wearing a Cast, Going to the Hospital, and *I Am, I Can, I Will,* Mr. Rogers' videocassettes, with guide. Family Communications, 4802 Fifth Ave., Pittsburgh, PA 15213.

FURTHER REFERENCES

Battle, Constance, "Chronic Physical Disease: Behavioral Aspects," *Pediatric Clinics of North America.* Vol. 22, No. 3:525–531, August 1975.

Benson, D. Frank and Dietrich Blumer, eds., *Psychiatric Aspects of Neurological Disease.* New York: Grune and Stratton, 1975.

Bermann, Thesi and Anna Freud, *Children in the Hospital.* New York: International University Press, 1965.

Borman, Leonard and others, *Helping People to Help Themselves: Prevention in Human Services,* Vol. 1, No. 3. New York: Haworth Press, Spring 1982.

Bowlby, John, *Separation.* New York: Basic Books, 1973.

Brewster, Arlene, "Chronically Ill Hospitalized Children's Concepts of Their Illness," *Pediatrics,* Vol. 69, No. 3, March 1982.

Burton, Lindy, *The Family Life of Sick Children: A Study of Families Coping with Chronic Childhood Disease.* London: Routledge and Kegan Paul, 1975.

Fedio, Paul and A. Mirsky, "Selective Intellectual Deficits in Children with Temporal Lobe or Centrencephalic Epilepsy," *Neuropsychologia,* Vol. 7, 287–300, 1969.

Fields, Grace, "Social Implications of Long-term Illness in Children" in *The Child with Disabling Illness* 2nd ed., eds. John A. Downey and Niels L. Low. New York: Raven Press, 1982.

Friedman, Stanford and others, "Behavioral Observations on Parents Anticipating the Death of a Child" in *Stress and Coping,* eds. Alan Monat and Richard S. Lazarus. New York: Columbia University Press, 1977.

Gardner, Richard A., "The Guilt Reaction of Parents of Children with Severe Physical Disease," *American Journal of Psychiatry,* 126:82, 1969.

Gliedman, John and William Roth, *The Unexpected Minority: Handicapped Children in America.* New York: The Carnegie Corporation, 1980.

Ilg, Frances and others, *School Readiness,* rev. ed. New York: Harper and Row, 1978.

Jackson, Gregg, "The Research Evidence on the Effects of Grade Retention," *Review of Educational Research,* Vol. 45, No. 4, 613–635, Fall 1975.

Jansky, Jeannette and Katrina DeHirsch, *Preventing Reading Failure.* New York: Harper and Row, 1972.

Johnson, Suzanne, "Psychosocial Factors in Juvenile Diabetes: A Review," *Journal of Behavioral Medicine,* Vol. 3, No. 1, 95–116, 1980.

Jurko, M. F. and O. J. Andy, "Verbal Learning Dysfunction with Combined Centre, Median and Amygdala Lesions," *Journal of Neurology, Neurosurgery and Psychiatry.* 40:695–698, 1977.

Langford, William S., "Child in Pediatric Hospital: Adaptation to Hospital and Illness," *American Journal of Orthopsychiatry,* 31:667–684, 1961.

Lazarus, Richard S., interviewed by Daniel Goleman, "Positive Denial, The Case For Not Facing Reality," *Psychology Today,* pp. 44–60, November 1979.

Linde, Leonard and others, "Attitudinal Factors in Congenital Heart Disease," *Pediatrics,* 38:92–101, 1966.

Lishman, W. A., *Organic Psychiatry: The Psychological Consequences of Cerebral Disorder.* Oxford, England: Blackwell Scientific Publications, 1978.

Madden, N. and J. Terrizzi and S. Friedman, "Psychological Issues in Mothers of Children with Hemophilia," *Developmental and Behavioral Pediatrics,* Vol. 3, No. 3, September 1982.

Magrab, Phyllis, ed., *Psychological Management of Pediatric Problems,* Vol. I. Baltimore: University Park Press, 1978.

Mason, Edward A., "The Hospitalized Child: His Emotional Needs," *New England Journal of Medicine,* 272:406, 1965.

Mattson, Ake, "Social and Behavioral Studies on Hemophiliac Children and Their Families," *Journal of Pediatrics,* 68:952, 1966.

Mazzullo, Mariann and Beatrice Jacobson, "Education of the Physically Handicapped Child" in *The Child with Disabling Illness* 2nd ed., eds. John A. Downey and Niels L. Low. New York: Raven Press, 1982.

Mungus, Dan, "Interictal Behavior Abnormality in Temporal Lobe Epilepsy," *Archives of General Psychiatry,* 39:108–111, January 1982.

Nott, Deborah and Phyllis Yeager, "Mainstreaming: Does the Regular Educator View the Process Differently than the Special Educator?" *The Directive Teacher,* Vol. 2, No. 2, Fall 1979.

Pincus, Jonathan and Gary S. Tucker, *Behavioral Neurology.* 2nd ed. London: Oxford University Press, 1978.

Pless, Ivan B., and Klaus J. Roghmann, "Chronic Illness and Its Consequences: Observations Based on Three Epidemiologic Surveys," *Journal of Pediatrics,* Vol. 79, 3:351–359, September 1971.

Pless, Ivan B. and P. Pinkerton, *Chronic Childhood Disorders: Promoting Patterns of Adjustment.* London: Henry Kimpton, 1975.

Schoenberg, Bernard and others, eds., *Anticipatory Grief.* New York: Columbia University Press, 1974.

Schaffer, David, "Psychiatric Aspects of Brain Injury in Childhood," *Developmental Medicine and Child Neurology.* 15:211–220, 1973.

Silverstein, Roger, "Learning Problems as a Symptom of Family Dysfunction," Journal of the Association for the Care of Children's Health, Vol. 9, No. 4, 122–125, Spring 1981.

———— "The Critically Ill Child and Acute Marital Stress: Social Work Intervention." Paper presented at the First International Conference on Pediatric Social Work, August 14, 1982, Chicago, IL.

Stone, Robert, "Administration of Hospitals Caring for the Long-term Sick Child," in *The Child with Disabling Illness.* 2nd ed., eds. John A. Downey and Niels L. Low. New York: Raven Press, 1982.

Thornton, Susan and William K. Frankenburg, eds., *Child Health Care Communications.* Skillman, NJ: Johnson and Johnson Baby Products, Pediatric Round Table Series, 1983.

Trebles, Pat and Sandra McCormick and John Cooper, "Problems in Mainstreaming at the Grassroots," *The Directive Teacher,* Vol. 4, No. 2, Summer–Fall 1982.

Wilson, Robert, "Psychological Aspects of Epilepsy." Department of Psychology and Social Sciences, Rush Presbyterian-St. Luke's Medical Center, Chicago, IL.

INDEX

A

Abandonment, fear of. *See* Separation anxiety.
Advice, teachers and giving:
  child behavior and, 146, 183
  impending death and, 137–139
Anxiety, 29
  buddy system and, 30–31
  counseling and, 31
  effects of reducing, 128
  how a teacher should respond to children's, 42–43
  how to reduce, 129–130
  parents', 121–122, 127–129
  recognizing symptoms of, 30
  separation, 8–9
  See also Fears (children's).
Arthrogryposis, physical handicaps with, 22
Association for the Care of Children's Health (ACCH), 97
Asthma:
  caused by emotional factors, 61
  explanatory statement for, 52

B

Barriers:
  Child Study Evaluation and, 152
  doctor/teacher, 148–149
  overcoming, 144–146
  parental, 142–143
  teacher, 143
Behavior:
  home versus school, 145–146
  immature, 81–82
  siblings and negative, 112
Behavior disorders:
  organic origin of, 68–73
  psychological origin of, 67–68
Brain damage, effects on behavior, 71–72
Buddy system, anxiety and use of the, 30–31

C

Cerebral palsy:
  concealment and, 12

Cerebral palsy (*Cont'd*)
  emotional effects of, 65–66
  explanatory statement for, 52
  physical handicaps with, 21–22
Changes, physical:
  returning to school and, 100–101
Chemotherapy, explanatory statement for, 52
Child development/family history, Child Study Evaluation and, 169–170
Child-life program, 97
Child-life specialist, 97–98
Child Study Evaluation:
  child's doctor and, 151
  collating data from a, 174
  components of a, 168–174
  learning disabilities and use of, 76
  parental fears, 176–180
  special class placement and, 160
  teacher/parent roles in a, 174–176
  used to remove barriers, 152
Chores, self-esteem and the use of, 47
Chronically ill children, difference between handicapped children and, 21, 23–28
Classmates. *See* Peers.
Class placement:
  special, 160–164
  teachers and, 11–12
Competition, alternatives to:
  cooperative games as, 54–55
  individual sports as, 54
Complications and chronic illnesses, 26–27
Concealment of illness, how to deal with parents', 12–13
Conferences:
  parent-teacher, 144–145
  preentrance, 10
  with angry parents, 147–148
Coping:
  factors that contribute to successful, 127
  how parents can help children in, 129–130
  teacher's role when parents aren't, 138–139
Coping mechanisms:
  fantasy, 45–46
  magical thinking, 29
  older children's, 29
  role-playing, 28
  use of literature, 50

LS-8　　58　14858